Pre- and Post-Operative Services for the Amputee with Diabetes

What the health care provider needs to know to prepare and care for amputee patients

Sander Nassan, CPO, FAAOP
Editor

American Diabetes Association.

Cure • Care • Commitment®

Director, Book Publishing, Robert Anthony; *Managing Editor, Book Publishing*, Abe Ogden; *Acquisitions Editor, Professional Books*, Victor Van Beuren; *Production Manager*, Melissa Sprott; *Editor, Composition*, Aptara, Inc.; *Cover Design*, Koncept, Inc.; *Printer*, Worzalla Publishing.

Printed in the United States of America
1 3 5 7 9 10 8 6 4 2

The suggestions and information contained in this publication are generally consistent with the *Clinical Practice Recommendations* and other policies of the American Diabetes Association, but they do not represent the policy or position of the Association or any of its boards or committees. Reasonable steps have been taken to ensure the accuracy of the information presented. However, the American Diabetes Association cannot ensure the safety or efficacy of any product or service described in this publication. Individuals are advised to consult a physician or other appropriate health care professional before undertaking any diet or exercise program or taking any medication referred to in this publication. Professionals must use and apply their own professional judgment, experience, and training and should not rely solely on the information contained in this publication before prescribing any diet, exercise, or medication. The American Diabetes Association—its officers, directors, employees, volunteers, and members—assumes no responsibility or liability for personal or other injury, loss, or damage that may result from the suggestions or information in this publication.

⊗ The paper in this publication meets the requirements of the ANSI Standard Z39.48-1992 (permanence of paper).

ADA titles may be purchased for business or promotional use or for special sales. To purchase more than 50 copies of this book at a discount, or for custom editions of this book with your logo, contact Lee Romano Sequeira, Special Sales & Promotions, at the address below, or at LRomano@diabetes.org or 703-299-2046.

For all other inquiries, please call 1-800-DIABETES.

American Diabetes Association
1701 North Beauregard Street
Alexandria, Virginia 22311

Library of Congress Cataloging-in-Publication Data

Pre- and post-operative services for the amputee with diabetes : what the healthcare provider needs to know to prepare and care for amputee patients / Sander Nassan et al.
 p. ; cm.
 Includes bibliographical references and index.
 ISBN 978-1-58040-266-8 (alk. paper)
 1. Leg–Amputation. 2. Amputees–Rehabilitation. 3. Diabetics–Rehabilitation.
4. Diabetes–Complications. 5. Diabetics–Surgery. 6. Artificial legs. I. Nassan, Sander.
II. American Diabetes Association.
 [DNLM: 1. Diabetes Complications–surgery. 2. Amputation.
3. Perioperative Care–methods. 4. Prostheses and Implants. WK 835 P922 2007]
 RD560.P69 2007
 617.5′8–dc22
                                                                    2007011445

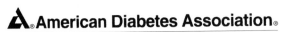

American Diabetes Association®
Cure • Care • Commitment®

Contents

Contributors

Sander Nassan, CPO, FAAOP, is a Clinical Prosthetist and Orthotist and owner of Prosthetic and Orthotic Associates in Scottsdale, Arizona. He is an adjunct faculty member in the Department of Chemical, Bio, and Materials Engineering at Arizona State University, and past chair of the Gait Society, a division of the American Academy of Orthotists and Prosthetists.

Jayer Chung, MD, is a Resident in Surgery and Research Fellow in the Department of Surgery at the University of Colorado Health Sciences Center in Denver, Colorado. His research interests include the effects of statin therapy on whole body energenics, the effects of peripheral arterial disease in skeletal muscle gene expression, and functional and technical outcomes after revascularization for critical limb ischemia.

Bertram E. Feingold, MD, FACS, FAAOS, lives in Scottsdale, Arizona where he has been in solo orthopedic surgery practice for 30 years. Active in the Scottsdale community, Dr. Feingold is on the staff of the Scottsdale Healthcare Osborn and Shea facilities.

David P. Guy, PT, MS, started his career as a physical therapist and clinical director for the United States Army. He was an associate professor of orthopedics and rehabilitation at Vanderbilt University, Nashville, Tennessee and is currently an outpatient physical therapist in the Scottsdale, Arizona area. An ardent volunteer, he has worked with numerous rehabilitation organizations, local, state, and federal agencies, and with various national and local disability advocacy organizations.

William R. Hiatt, MD, is the Novartis Foundation Endowed Professor for Cardiovascular Research in the Department of Medicine at the University of Colorado. He is currently Chief of the Section of Vascular Medicine and President of the Colorado Prevention Center for Cardiovascular Research. Active within the research and medical administrative communities, he is the current Chair of the Cardiovascular and Renal Drugs Advisory Committee for the Food and Drug Administration. His clinical research focuses on the epidemiology, pathophysiology, and treatment of peripheral arterial disease.

Steve McNamee, CP, worked with Prosthetics and Orthotics Associates in Scottsdale, Arizona as a clinician and branch facility manager. He currently is the owner of Artisan Prosthetics in Phoenix, Arizona. A skilled clinician, Mr. McNamee is very active in training prosthetic and orthotic professionals.

James Price, PhD, CPO, is President of Faith Prosthetic-Orthotic Services, Inc., a clinical practice specializing in artificial limb technology and orthopedic design based in Charlotte, North Carolina. His research interests include psychological issues in those who experience limb amputation and applied technology in prosthetic systems design.

Robert S. Schwartz, MD, is a Professor of Medicine/Geriatric Medicine and Head of the Division of Geriatric Medicine at the University of Colorado Health Sciences Center in Denver, Colorado. He also holds the position of Professor with the University of Washington School of Medicine, Division of Gerontology and Geriatric Medicine. His research interests range from geriatric medicine and gerontology to nutritional studies.

Stephanie A. Slayton, PT, DPT, CWS, is a Physical Therapist with the Pitt County Memorial Hospital in Greenville, North Carolina. She is a Certified Wound Care Specialist with the American Academy of Wound Management and is an adjunct faculty member of the Physical Therapy Department at East Carolina University.

Douglas Van Atta, CPO, practices prosthetics and orthotics in Cincinnati, Ohio. An active member of the American Academy of Orthotists and Prosthetists, he served on the AAOP Board of Directors for Region V and its Ohio Chapter. He also served on the Ohio Licensure Board for Orthotics, Prosthetics, and Pedorthics.

Dennis E. Weiland, MD, has practiced general and critical care surgery in Scottsdale, Arizona for 35 years. He is currently Director of Hyperbaric Medicine at Scottsdale Healthcare where he practices wound care and hyperbaric medicine and has published over 32 peer-reviewed articles. He is a Clinical Assistant Professor of Surgery at the University of Arizona where he taught surgery at the Maricopa Medical Center until 1998.

Tom Wolvos, MD, FACS, specializes in general and peripheral vascular surgery and practices general surgery, hyperbaric medicine, and advanced wound care at the Scottsdale Health Care Hospital and Wound Management Center. He is the founder of Scottsdale Surgical Consultants, P.C. and is the Medical Director of Scottsdale Healthcare Outpatient Wound Management Services.

Wesley N. Yamada, DPM, is chief of podiatry at Hu Hu Kam Memorial Hospital, in Sacaton, Arizona, located on the Gila River Reservation. He is a Diplomate with the American Board of Podiatric Surgery and a Fellow with both the American College of Foot and Ankle Surgeons and the American College of Foot Orthopedics and Medicine.

Preface

Each year more than 82,000 diabetes sufferers in North America alone are given the grim news that they need a partial foot or lower extremity amputation. Most find themselves in a panic situation, faced with thoughts of restricted mobility, a severely diminished lifestyle, and a genuine loss of self. What they typically find at the end of the process is greater mobility, more and healthier lifestyle options and a reengagement with life to their fullest extent. As a health care provider who works closely with diabetic patients, it is essential that you know and understand what your patient is facing when amputation becomes the only option. It is critical for you to know the numerous services available that will help your patient experience the desired outcome.

This book started as a conversation between Victor Van Beuren, Manager, Professional Book Acquisitions for the American Diabetes Association, and me. I argued against it, sure that what he was suggesting was readily available from another publisher. I was wrong. It was available from maybe five different sources and the tone of writing and the targeted readers were different from what Victor had in mind. So I agreed to take on this worthwhile project.

Our goal was to compile a book concerning the process and care that a new diabetic amputee would most likely experience. The authors have brought to light techniques and services available, and the clinicians who might best provide them to the diabetic amputee.

The writing is purposely accessible yet with a professional tone to inform primary care physicians, physician's assistants, and nurses as well as Certified Diabetes Educators (CDE). These dedicated professionals now have a single source concerning amputation, rehabilitation, and wound care. The chapters and subject matter can be easily referenced and ultimately shared with diabetic patients and their caregivers. The available information permits the diabetic educator to be better informed, thereby helping the patients and their families make the necessary quality-of-life decisions.

Our talented contributors were chosen because of their experience and dedication to the diabetic patient and the amputee. Three of our authors have not previously written for publication, but were up for the challenge. I was well aware of their records of exemplary patient care, and after several conversations with each, convinced them to sign on. I'm glad they did. Each author wrote from his or her humane and professional experience, thus providing us with a greater understanding of his or her specialty and personal philosophy. I congratulate and thank them for their very successful efforts.

As volume editor, I have personally benefited from reading and re-reading the chapters, and also by having wonderful discussions with the contributors. I am sure you, the reader, will appreciate the dedication and knowledge inherent in each chapter.

Two of the most repeated principles on good patient care were explicit communication and a team approach. I encourage you to learn who your patients' professional caregivers are and speak with them, ask questions, and encourage pro-patient discussions. The knowledge that you have of your patient's unique situations is of great interest to his or her prosthetist and physical therapist. Remember—everyone has the same goal of quality patient care and service.

I wish to give a very special thank you to my invaluable assistants Angie Wilson and Lana Nassan. Their on-time and on-target communications have kept this project on task.

Our desire is that this book adds to your knowledge about amputations, follow-up care, and the professionals who provide these services. This aspiration is met when you are better able to provide more thorough education and support for your patients.

Thanks for all you do and keep up the good work!

Sander Nassan, CPO, FAAOP
December 2006

Introduction

This book is set up to lead you through the choices and outcomes of surgery on to the immediate post-op process and then the prosthetic options.

The preferred outcome of managing the diabetic patient is compliance on his or her part and the avoidance of amputation. The statistics and parameters presented by Drs. Chung, Schwartz, and Hiatt keep us in the "here and now." Without using the big scary numbers that help raise consciousness and funds, this chapter gives us some sobering statistics concerning the very real people we are serving. These figures should impress us and motivate us to create programs and systems to better educate and protect our diabetic patient, with the goal to lower the current statistics.

And though we are working to maintain the education and health of our patients, the insidiousness of the disease demands a variety of wound care modalities to stay the decision to amputate. Stephanie Slayton, DPT, has contributed a comprehensive review of available wound care techniques. Dr. Slayton wrote from the perspective of saving the diabetic limb. These modalities and principles apply to healing and saving the residuum and of course the contralateral lower extremity. Her thoroughness provides the primary physician and Certified Diabetes Educator with a menu of modalities to refer to and learn about, all in the sprit of enhancing the discussion with a wound care specialist and supporting your patient during the healing process.

If these prove unsuccessful, then life-saving amputations will need to be performed. Please realize that the wound care modalities available prior to amputation are often needed postsurgically.

Surgeons Yamada and Feingold provide us with an overview of partial foot amputations and major lower extremity amputations. Dr. Yamada speaks to us about how disruptive amputation can be to the mechanical balance of the foot. He also generously shares some of the orthotic and prosthetic options for managing a partial foot amputation.

All of us take the foot for granted. It is remarkable structure. Think of this later—as you walk to your car. Every time your heel hits the ground, the force is 20% greater than your body weight. Not the imagined half of your weight, but 1.2 times your entire weight! This multiple increases in relation to how aggressive you are walking. Jogging and running are even more forceful, often reaching 6 times body weight!

Dr. Feingold gently presents the subject of major amputations of the leg. His contribution introduces us to the four common sites (levels) of amputation between the hip and ankle and the criteria used to determine each level.

Drs. Dennis E. Weiland and Thomas Wolvos, whom I refer to as the "Push and Pull" of wound care, expand on the wound healing techniques of hyperbaric treatment and vacuum assisted closure, respectively. Their experience and success are evident, making their thoughtful contributions accessible and informative.

As things go, amputation is often the procedure necessary to preserve life and improve the quality of that life. Which is where my mentor and friend Doug Van Atta, CPO, chimes in. His decades of service and dedication to the amputee (diabetic or otherwise) will be immediately evident to you. Doug starts with the ideal situation of having a prosthetist meet with the patient and family if possible before surgery. This meeting assures the person that there is a professional who spends his or her entire day solving problems for people without limbs. This is reassuring to the patient. Also, the prosthetist is not a new face after amputation, but rather a familiar and friendly one with answers to the scores of questions relating to the prostheses and rehabilitation. Doug also covers the options of immediate postoperative prosthetic care.

You will find that proper postop care permits on-time and even early discharge from the hospital, and shortens the time between amputation and the initial prosthetic fitting. This is important stuff!!

Doug's contributions are followed by another teacher of mine—David Guy, MS, PT. David is a true patient advocate, pushing the doctors and prosthetists to provide the best outcome for their patients. All the while, he is coaxing the most from his patients. David is a proponent of early intervention with new amputees. His goal is to improve balance and strength while protecting the contralateral leg and residuum. I encourage you to seek out a physical therapist who is well versed in wound care, gait, and the prosthetic process, and who communicates well.

Steve McNamee, CP, and I had the pleasure of working together for several years. I was always impressed by his thoughtfulness and thoroughness when it came to prosthetic patient care. His discussion of prosthetic options for your patients is clear and easy to follow, his images help the cause. You will especially appreciate his "pearls," which are important to keep in mind. There are almost too many choices in prosthetic feet, knees, suspension systems, socket shapes, materials, and cosmetic finishes for anyone not professionally involved to be familiar, let alone comfortable, with. Steve's pearls will help you see past some of the clutter (and expense) to appreciate a prosthesis that meets the daily needs and lifestyle of your patient. The prosthesis should neither restrict an amputee nor consist of componentry that is beyond the amputee's capabilities.

Our final chapter is by James Price, PhD, CPO. He shares with us the psychosocial and psychophysiological manifestations of amputation and phantom limb phenomena. The psychosocial cost of amputation is thoroughly covered by Dr. Price. This contribution is a valuable source to help us understand and support the new (diabetic) amputee. We also benefit from Dr. Price's discussion on phantom limb and pain. Phantom limb sensation is a distinct phenomenon from pain and must be presented as such when talking to the amputee patients and their families. Since phantom limb occurs in nearly 100% in new amputees, the goal is to ward off the onset of phantom pain or prevent it from becoming a chronic pain condition. Dr. Price's insights into the psychology and various learning styles of the amputee patient help us to provide holistic care and support to our patients. This thoughtful contribution rounds out this book, which, until now has been decidedly physical.

I once again want to emphasize the team approach to successful amputation, wound care, and rehabilitation. The goal of this publication is to provide a foundation of information in the various specialties that affect successful amputation and prosthetic outcomes. My wish is that you utilize this resource to initiate and continue conversations that lead to better care and a return to a satisfying quality of life for the new diabetic amputee.

In closing, I suggest that a new amputee seek out a support group. Some are independent groups—most are organized by a hospital or rehabilitation facility.

The Amputee Coalition of America (ACA) is a great resource and the one that I guide my own patients to.

Amputee Coalition of America (ACA)
900 E. Hill Ave., Ste 285
Knoxville, KN 37915
www.amputee-coalition.org
888-267-5669

Sander Nassan, CPO, FAAOP
December 2006

1

Diabetes Mellitus and Peripheral Arterial Disease

Jayer Chung, MD
Robert S. Schwartz, MD
William R. Hiatt, MD

Introduction

Peripheral arterial disease (PAD) is one of the major manifestations of systemic atherosclerosis, where the perfusion of the lower extremities is compromised due to occlusions of the vessel lumen. There are two clinical syndromes: intermittent claudication (IC) and critical limb ischemia (CLI). IC occurs when atherosclerotic plaque limits the perfusion of a patient's leg, causing disabling muscle cramping of the calf or thigh with minimal exercise. This symptom is very reproducible and is relieved by rest. Patients with more severe plaque burden and further limitation in the perfusion to the lower limb can present with CLI, complaining of leg pain at rest and/or ischemic ulcerations (Luscher et al. 2003).

Due to the systemic nature of atherosclerosis, there is a strong overlap between PAD and other atherosclerotic disease processes such as coronary artery disease (CAD) and cerebrovascular accidents (CVA). The annual rate of myocardial infarction (MI), stroke, and vascular death in patients with PAD is 5% to 6% annually. The presence of diabetes worsens both the incidence and severity of the manifestations of atherosclerosis. For patients with unstable angina, diabetes increases mortality by 57%. Stroke risk is similarly increased, with a threefold increase risk of stroke among patients taking hypoglycemic agents compared to nondiabetics (Luscher et al. 2003).

The incidence and prevalence of diabetes mellitus is increasing in Western populations (Muller et al. 2002), likely due to sedentary lifestyle patterns that contribute to obesity and insulin resistance (Diehm et al. 2006). Diabetes increases both the incidence and severity of ischemia to the lower extremities two- to fourfold (Luscher et al. 2003). The incidence of PAD is also increasing due to the aging of the U.S. population, and the greater incidence and prevalence of diabetes and other atherosclerotic risk factors associated with aging. The presence of both diabetes and lower limb arterial disease markedly increases a patient's risk of developing ischemic ulceration and subsequent amputation. Moreover, the clinical expression of PAD in diabetics is more virulent, with increased presence of infrageniculate plaques and calcification in the medial layer of blood vessels (Luscher et al. 2003; Diehm et al. 2006). The infrageniculate distribution of disease portends an increased risk of subsequent amputation due to the paucity of options for collateral vessel development and revascularization (Luscher et al. 2003; Faglia et al. 1998). Over the past decade, there has been an increase in the number of amputations performed for limbs with arterial disease in diabetic patients (Dillingham et al. 2005). Diabetics have an eight- to twelve-fold increased risk of lower extremity amputation. In published studies, the annual incidence is approximately 5–8 amputations per 1,000 diabetic patients (.5%–.8%) (Diehm et al. 2006; Hamalainen et al. 1999; Morris et al. 1998). This includes minor amputations (digital, partial foot) and major amputations (below the knee, and above the knee).

The risk of subsequent re-amputation and of mortality is worse among diabetics undergoing an amputation for critical limb ischemia. The 1-, 3-, and 5-year mortality rates after an initial amputation have been reported to be as high as 15%, 38%, and 68%, respectively, in diabetic patients (Larsson et al. 1998). Re-amputation rates after a first index amputation range from 14% to 34% at 1 year in this group (Dillingham et al. 2005; Larsson et al. 1998). The 3- and 5-year re-amputation rates are 30% and 49%, respectively.

As expected, the type of amputation plays a role in subsequent functional ability. Larsson et al. (1998) demonstrated that independent living status was more often preserved in patients with minor pedal amputations compared with those undergoing major amputations (93% versus 61%, respectively). Health-related quality of life is also markedly worse among this subgroup of diabetics (Ragnarson Tennval et al. 2000). Wound healing occurred at a median of 29 weeks for minor amputations, and 8 weeks with a major amputation. Major amputations heal more quickly than minor amputations due to the richer blood supply proximally, with above-knee amputations healing more rapidly than below-knee amputations (Ragnarson-Tennval et al. 2000; Nehler et al. 2003). The number of diabetics retaining the ability to ambulate 1 km after an index amputation is 70% for minor amputees but only 19% for major amputees. Only 52% of diabetics utilize a prosthesis after healed amputations (Larsson et al. 1998). From 1996–1997, Medicare costs for amputees with diabetes exceeded $4.3 billion (Dillingham et al. 2005).

Due to the poor technical, functional, and quality-of-life outcomes after amputation for diabetics, it is imperative that primary care providers are aware of the peripheral vascular status of their diabetic patients. Unfortunately, there is evidence of inadequate awareness of PAD among primary care physicians (McLafferty et al. 2000), inadequately aggressive risk factor modification, and slow referral to vascular surgeons (Lange et al. 2004; Hirsch et al. 2001). These factors probably significantly increase the severity of disease at presentation to the vascular surgeon, the likelihood for amputation, and its attendant morbidity and mortality. With the expected rise in the incidence of diabetes and PAD, appropriate awareness of the referring physician becomes increasingly important. This chapter will focus on the diagnosis and treatment of patients with PAD, highlighting the diagnostic and therapeutic challenges unique to the diabetic population.

Diagnosis

The diagnosis of PAD is usually established by the measurement of blood pressures in the lower extremity. From a clinical perspective, the most salient features of the diagnosis, however, are the history, physical examination, and noninvasive vascular measurements. Classically, patients with IC present with exertional leg pain relieved with rest. The pain is typically described as crampy in nature, localizing to the calf or thigh. Patients with CLI complain of rest pain and/or ulcers that fail to heal after an adequate period of time (2 weeks). This is associated with a decrement or loss of pulses in the femoral, popliteal, or pedal regions. Ankle-brachial indices (ABI) are also decreased (<0.90) in the symptomatic limb (Townsend et al. 2004).

ABIs are obtained by measuring the systolic blood pressure from bilateral brachial arteries, dorsalis pedis, and posterior tibial arteries using a handheld Doppler ultrasound and a blood pressure cuff. The brachial systolic pressure that is used is the highest recorded from either arm. The ankle pressure that is used is the highest pressure obtained for each limb among the posterior tibial and dorsalis pedis arteries. The ABI is then calculated as follows: ankle systolic pressure divided by brachial systolic pressure. Normal ABIs are between 0.9 and 1.3. Values of less than 0.9 indicate a deficit in lower limb perfusion. Values greater than 1.3 are considered to be supra-systolic (Townsend et al. 2004).

The differential diagnosis for IC symptoms includes spinal stenosis, venous claudication, chronic compartment syndrome, nerve root compression, and Baker's cyst. These differ from IC in that they are all relieved with elevation of the limb or change in body position. Of these, spinal stenosis (also called pseudo-claudication) may be the most difficult to discern from IC. It, too, is associated with exertion and can be quite reproducible. However, pain from spinal stenosis often occurs while standing at rest and can be quickly relieved with spinal flexion (e.g., walking while bending over a shopping cart). Arthritis can also cause pain in the leg, although the onset and relief of the pain is usually more variable; conversely, the onset and resolution of pain in IC classically occurs after a consistent amount of exercise, and resolves with a consistent amount of rest (Townsend et al. 2004).

Diabetics often have concurrent pathophysiological processes that further confound the diagnosis of PAD. Medial arterial calcification is common in diabetics, causing false elevations in the patients' ABI (a false-negative test). Diabetic neuropathy may also result in no (anesthesia) or abnormal (dysesthesia) sensation in the affected limb, limiting the sensation of claudication, or rest pain. Mal perforans ulcers result from the absence of pain sensation at the pressure points of the foot, resulting in painless ulcerations. These ulcers may be treated incorrectly when the ischemic component of the ulcer's etiology is underestimated or overlooked.

In the presence of medial arterial calcification and falsely elevated ABI (>1.3), the utilization of toe pressures is essential (Townsend et al. 2004; Brooks et al. 2001). The toe pressure and toe-brachial index are key to quantifying the degree of ischemia in the affected limb. Toe pressures less than 50 mm Hg are considered an indication for angiography and possible surgical or interventional therapy to improve perfusion to the limb. Toe pressures are obtained by using a small cuff that can occlude the blood flow to the great toe, and using photoplethysmography to estimate blood flow and hence pressure in the digit (Townsend et al. 2004; Brooks et al. 2001). The utility of toe pressures is limited to patients with falsely elevated ABIs, as toe pressure measurements in diabetics with normal or decreased ABIs have failed to improve the sensitivity of diagnosing PAD (Brooks et al. 2001). Hence, toe pressure measurements should be limited to those with evidence of medial arterial calcification.

Diabetics with atypical symptoms of IC represent a unique diagnostic challenge. These patients can have normal ABIs and toe pressures, and complain of pain with uncharacteristic features or in unusual locations. For these patients, a thorough history and physical examination is still essential to rule out nonatherosclerosis-related causes of pain. Exercise testing can be helpful in ascertaining whether there is an ischemic component to the patient's clinical appearance (Townsend et al. 2004). Patients with symptomatic PAD but normal ABIs may show a decrement of the ABI with the treadmill exercise test, thereby confirming the diagnosis. However, the patient must be sufficiently fit to tolerate a graded exercise treadmill examination.

The ischemic component to a diabetic ulceration is often overlooked, because a large proportion of these ulcerations are primarily neuropathic in etiology. However, two recent studies show that the prevalence of ischemia in diabetics presenting with ulceration to be as high as 45% (Campbell et al. 2000; Moulik et al. 2003). Therefore, all patients with a history of diabetes presenting with pedal ulceration should undergo a full vascular evaluation with ABI measurement (toe pressures if applicable). Early consultation with a vascular surgeon is essential to prevent the further progression to pedal necrosis.

Angiography is used to localize the atherosclerotic plaques, and to assess whether they are amenable to repair (percutaneous or open). Angiography should not be used to diagnose PAD. This is because traditional angiography is an invasive procedure with a 1% to 3% complication rate (Townsend et al. 2004). Magnetic resonance angiography (MRA) is being utilized with increased frequency, though the cost and limited availability prohibits its use as a first-line diagnostic test. MRA should be used in patients who have contraindications to conventional angiography. Select patients with discrete atherosclerotic lesions easily amenable to open bypass are also receiving MRA to avoid the complications associated with conventional angiography. Because MRA has been shown to have poorer resolution of the distal tibial and pedal vasculature, conventional angiography has remained the gold standard for evaluating PAD, especially in diabetic patients. However, with improving technology and radiologist familiarity with MRA interpretation, MRA may soon supplant conventional angiography as the diagnostic study of choice among diabetics with PAD (Kreitner et al. 2000).

Treatment

Nonsurgical Therapy

Nonsurgical interventions are reserved for patients with mild-to-moderate IC. Education regarding the importance of aggressive risk factor management and optimal foot care is essential for diabetics and their caregivers. Studies show that 10% of all patients over the age of 70 have symptoms of IC, and more than half of these consider the symptoms to be a part of "normal" aging (McLafferty et al. 2000). Primary care physicians frequently lack sufficient awareness of PAD risk among diabetics, leading to suboptimal management of risk factors and delays in initial diagnosis (McLafferty et al. 2000; Lange et al. 2004; Hirsch et al. 2001). Frequent podiatric follow-up, proper orthoses, and improved patient education have all been shown to decrease the rates of new ulceration, recurrent ulceration, and amputation among diabetics (Faglia et al. 2001; Tentolouris et al. 2004).

Screening of all diabetics and other at-risk patients with ABI measurements can improve the detection of previously undiagnosed PAD and enhance treatment.

Aggressive medical management of hypertension, smoking, and dyslipidemia are necessary to optimally manage a patient with PAD due to the systemic nature of atherosclerotic disease. Prevention of progression of PAD and other cardiovascular events should be the goal of the primary care physician. Optimal medical management can reduce the risk of cardiovascular events among diabetics by approximately 50% (Luscher et al. 2003). In addition to diet modification and smoking cessation, medications such as statins, ACE-inhibitors, and beta-blockers are critical to decreasing the risk of disease progression. Current National Cholesterol Education Program (NCEP) and American Diabetes Association (ADA) recommended targets for low density lipoprotein (LDL) are <100 mg/dL, HDL >45 mg/dL, total cholesterol <185 mg/dL, and triglycerides <150 mg/dL. More recent evidence suggests that lowering LDL cholesterol even further provides more of a protective benefit (Haffner 2005; Skrha et al. 2005). Blood pressure is recommended to be <130/80 mm/Hg. The target for HbA1c is <7.0% (Skrha et al. 2005). Although there is an epidemiological link between diabetes and the development of PAD, strict glycemic control has been shown to provide little if any benefit in reducing the risk of stroke, amputation, or death (Luscher et al. 2003).

For patients with claudication, there is a growing body of evidence that exercise therapy can significantly improve functional status and quality of life. Health-related questionnaire scores are also improved with exercise. The biochemical pathways by which claudication is improved with exercise are unclear, but are presently being investigated. Supervised exercise therapy appears to be superior to home-based programs. Maintenance of exercise therapy is required for the maintenance of improved walking distance and claudication time (Menard et al. 2004).

There are two drugs that have been U.S. Food and Drug Administration-approved for the treatment of claudication: pentoxifylline and cilostazol, with the latter being shown to be more effective. Cilostazol, at dosages of 50–100 mg by mouth twice per day has been shown to improve peak walking distances in prospective randomized clinical trials (Beebe et al. 1999). It improves peak walking distances and claudication times compared to pentoxifylline and placebo (Dawson et al. 2000). Cilostazol is a type III phosphodiesterase inhibitor that increases cAMP levels in both smooth muscle and platelets, resulting in vascular smooth muscle cell relaxation, and decreased platelet aggregation. Cilostazol has been shown to be 10–30 times more effective at inhibiting platelet aggregation than aspirin or ticlopidine. The specific mechanisms of action remain unclear (Beebe et al. 1999; Dawson et al. 2000). Patients with PAD and congestive heart failure (CHF) should not take cilostazol due to the potential concern of increasing mortality.

The role of antiplatelet therapy in PAD is critical in reducing the risk of systemic events. In patients with PAD and other evidence of cardiovascular disease (prior MI or stroke), aspirin should be prescribed. Clopidogrel is also approved as an antiplatelet drug for PAD and it may be more effective than aspirin based on a subgroup analysis from the CAPRIE trial (CAPRIE Steering Committee 1996). Future studies will further clarify the role of antiplatelet therapy in PAD, though at present it is recommended that anti-platelet therapy be implemented in all patients with diabetes and PAD (Luscher et al. 2003; CAPRIE Steering Committee 1996).

Surgical Therapy

There are three main surgical therapies for patients with PAD: endovascular, open surgical bypass, or amputation. Overall, there is evidence to show that diabetes independently predicts poorer outcomes, with higher rates of subsequent amputation, re-stenosis/graft occlusion, perioperative morbidity, and mortality (Luscher et al. 2003; Auvivola et al. 2004; Calle-Pascual et al. 2001). There are no unique indications for revascularization for diabetics, with critical limb ischemia, or short-distance (<150 feet) claudication being the usual indications for revascularization. There are no widely accepted guidelines to dictate which patients undergo primary amputation, conservative therapy, percutaneous therapy, open surgical therapy, or some other combination of these therapies. This is an area actively being investigated in vascular surgery (Kalbaugh et al. 2004). The most appropriate surgical therapy is dependent on the patients' co-morbidities, preoperative ambulatory and living status, technical feasibility to repair the lesions, the degree of pedal necrosis, surgeon preference, and the patient's own wishes (Hirsch et al. 2001; Kalbaugh et al. 2004; Atar et al. 2005). Therefore, the surgical therapy chosen is highly individualized.

Endovascular therapies (percutaneous transluminal angioplasty +/− stenting) in CLI and short-distance claudication have proven to be technically feasible and safe, with comparable outcomes to open surgical endarterectomy/bypass (Atar et al. 2005; Kudo et al. 2005; Feiring et al. 2004). The technical results are also comparable among diabetic and nondiabetic CLI patients, with 5-year primary patency rates of 88%, with 1.7% of patients undergoing a subsequent major amputation (Faglia et al. 2005). Data on functional outcomes, health-related quality-of-life measures, and long-term results after primary endovascular therapy are still needed, as well as comparisons with non-operative and open surgical therapies for revascularization. Early results, however, appear to indicate that primary endovascular therapy for CLI in diabetics is a safe and feasible procedure, with similar technical success as open surgery. Percutaneous therapy is generally reserved for patients with lesions technically amenable to endovascular repair, and/or has severe medical co-morbidities preventing the safe application of general anesthesia. Patients who also have no technical options for open surgical therapy (such as lack of venous conduit), or who have had multiple operations in the leg preventing a safe open surgical operation also often undergo endovascular therapy (Hirsch et al. 2001; Kalbaugh et al. 2004).

Open surgical bypass is the gold standard of therapy for revascularizing chronically ischemic limbs in both diabetics and nondiabetics. It is chosen due to its proven durability and success (Townsend et al. 2004). When compared to nondiabetics, diabetics are more likely to undergo distal revascularizations. They were also more likely to undergo simultaneous partial-foot amputation, and have wound complications. Diabetics with CLI have lower 3-year graft patency and limb salvage rates relative to nondiabetics (Calle-Pascual et al. 2001). Diabetes has also been shown to independently predict poor wound healing after infrainguinal bypass (Goshima et al. 2004). Functional outcomes and health-related quality of life have not been consistently related to the presence of diabetes. One can infer, however, because diabetics have prolonged healing and ulcerations, both of which correlate with lower health-related quality-of-life scores (Ragnarson-Tennval et al. 2000), that they would have a lower quality-of-life ratings after infrainguinal bypass.

Diabetics with CLI and minor or major lower extremity amputation suffer poorer outcomes. The ulcer recurrence rate in diabetics after amputation is 23%–30% at 5 years (Diehm 2006; Hamalainen et al. 1999; Larsson et al. 1998). Patients with an index minor versus major amputation have no difference in subsequent amputation rates. However, diabetics in both groups of patients suffered from lower rates of return to preoperative ambulatory and living status (Larsson et al. 1998). Mortality is also worse for diabetics undergoing amputation rather than revascularization for CLI (Calle-Pascual et al. 2001). Prevention of further ulceration with frequent physician visits, proper orthoses, and patient education have been shown to improve recurrent ulcer rates after minor amputations (Dalla Paola et al. 2003). It is clear, however, that diabetics undergoing amputation for CLI have the worst outcomes with respect to mortality, recurrent ulceration, subsequent re-amputation, and infection when compared to nondiabetic populations. In general, primary amputation is reserved for patients who do not have the ability to ambulate preoperatively. Patients who have septic lesions in the lower extremities, or extensive pedal lesions that will not permit the reconstruction of a functional foot, also frequently undergo primary amputation (Hirsch et al. 2001; Kalbaugh et al. 2004).

Conclusions

Diabetes affects approximately 100 million people worldwide, with the prevalence expected to increase substantially as rates of obesity increase (Diehm et al. 2006). The prevalence of PAD is also expected to rise as the population ages with 8–12 million patients in the United States already affected (Skrha et al. 2005). Diabetes is presently the number one cause of nontraumatic limb amputations in the United States, with the number of cases on the rise (Diehm et al. 2006). Due to the high morbidity and mortality these amputees sustain, emphasis must be placed on prevention through patient and primary caregiver education. Hopefully, improved control of medical risk factors, greater awareness of the risks and dangers of limb loss, and earlier referral to vascular specialists will produce a decline in the need for amputation and possibly improve outcomes after revascularization.

References

Atar E, Siegel Y, Avrahami R, Bartal G, Bachar GN, Belenky A. Balloon angioplasty of popliteal and crural arteries in elderly with critical chronic limb ischemia. *Eur J Radiol* 53:287–292, 2005.

Aulivola B, Hile CN, Hamdan AD, Sheahan MG, Veraldi JR, Skillman JJ, Campbell DR, Scovell SD, LoGerfo FW, Pomposelli FB Jr. Major lower extremity amputation: Outcome of a modern series. *Arch Surg* 139:395–399, 2004.

Beebe HG, Dawson DL, Cutler BS, Herd JA, Strandness DE Jr, Bortey EB, Forbes WP. A New pharmacological treatment for intermittent claudication. *Arch Intern Med* 159:2041–2050, 1999.

Brooks B, Dean R, Patel S, Wu B, Molyneaux L, Yue DK. TBI or not TBI: That is the question. Is it better to measure toe pressure than ankle pressure in diabetic patients? *Diabet Med* 18:528–532, 2001.

Calle-Pascual AL, Duran A, Diaz A, Monux G, Serrano FJ, de la Torre NG, Moraga I, Calle JR, Charro A, Maranes JP. Comparison of peripheral arterial reconstruction in diabetic and non-diabetic patients: A prospective clinic-based study. *Diabetes Res Clin Prac* 53:129–136, 2001.

Campbell WB, Ponette D, Sugiono M. Long-term results following operation for diabetic foot problems: Arterial disease confers a poor prognosis. *Eur J Vasc Endovasc Surg* 19:174–177, 2000.

CAPRIE Steering Committee. A randomised, blinded, trial of clopidogrel versus aspirin in patients at risk of ischaemic events (CAPRIE). *Lancet* 348:1329–1339, 1996.

Dalla Paola L, Faglia E, Caminiti M, Clerici G, Ninkovic S, Deanesi V. Ulcer recurrence following first ray amputation in diabetic patients: A cohort prospective study. *Diabetes Care* 26(6):1874–1878, 2003.

Dawson DL, Cutler BS, Hiatt WR, Hobson RW 2nd, Martin JD, Bortey EB, Forbes WP, Strandness DE Jr. A comparison of cilostazol and pentoxifylline for treating intermittent claudication. *Am J Med* 109:523–530, 2000.

Diehm N, Shang A, Silvestro A, Do DD, Dick F, Schmidli J, Mahler F, Baumgartner I. Association of cardiovascular risk factors with pattern of lower limb atherosclerosis in 2,659 patients undergoing angioplasty. *Eur J Vasc Endovasc Surg* 31:59–63, 2006.

Dillingham TR, Pezzin LE, Shore AD. Reamputation, mortality, and health care costs among persons with dysvascular lower-limb amputations. *Arch Phys Med Rehabil* 86:480–486, 2005.

Faglia E, Favales F, Quarantiello A, Calia P, Clelia P, Brambilla G, Rampoldi A, Morabito A. Angiographic evaluation of peripheral arterial occlusive disease and its role as a prognostic determinant for major amputation in diabetic subjects with foot ulcers. *Diabetes Care* 21(4):625–630, 1998.

Faglia E, Favales F, Morabito A. New ulceration, new major amputation, and survival rates in diabetic subjects hospitalized for foot ulceration from 1990 to 1993. *Diabetes Care* 24(1):78–83, 2001.

Faglia E, Dalla Paola L, Clerici G, Clerissi J, Graziani L, Fusaro M, Gabrielli L, Losa S, Stella A, Gargiulo M, Mantero M, Caminiti M, Ninkovic S, Curci V, Morabito A. Peripheral angioplasty as the first-choice revascularization procedure in diabetic patients with critical limb ischemia: Prospective study of 993 consecutive patients hospitalized and followed between 1999 and 2003. *Eur J Vasc Endovasc Surg* 29:620–627, 2005.

Feiring AJ, Wesolowski AA, Lade S. Primary stent-supported angioplasty for the treatment of below-knee critical limb ischemia and severe claudication: Early and one-year outcomes. *J Am Coll Cardiol* 44:2307–2314, 2004.

Goshima KR, Mills JL Sr, Hughes JD. A new look at outcomes after infrainguinal bypass surgery: Traditional reporting standards underestimate the expenditure of effort required to attain limb salvage. *J Vasc Surg* 39(2):330–335, 2004.

Haffner S. Rationale for new American Diabetes Association guidelines: Are national cholesterol education program goals adequate for the patient with diabetes mellitus? *Am J Cardiol* 96[suppl]:33E–36E, 2005.

Hamalainen H, Ronnemaa T, Halonen JP, Toikka T. Factors predicting lower extremity amputation in patients with type 1 or type 2 diabetes mellitus: A population-based 7-year follow-up study. *J Intern Med* 246:97–103, 1999.

Hirsch AT, Criqui MH, Treat-Jacobson D, Regensteiner JG, Creager MA, Olin JW, Krook SH, Hunninghake DB, Comerota AJ, Walsh ME, McDermott MM, Hiatt WR. Peripheral arterial disease detection, awareness, and treatment in primary care. *JAMA* 286(11):1317–1324, 2001.

Kalbaugh CA, Taylor SM, Cull DL, Blackhurst DW, Gray BH, Langan EM 3rd, Dellinger MB, McClary GE Jr, Jackson MR, Carsten CG 3rd, Snyder BA, York JW, Youkey JR. Invasive treatment of chronic limb ischemia according to the Lower Extremity Grading System (LEGS) Score: A 6-month report. *J Vasc Surg* 39:1268–1276, 2004.

Kreitner KF, Kalden P, Neufang A, Duber C, Krummenauer F, Kustner E, Laub G, Thelen M. Diabetes and peripheral arterial occlusive disease: Prospective comparison of 3-dimensional MR angiography with conventional digital subtraction. *Am J Roentgenol* 174:171–179, 2000.

Kudo T, Chandra FA, Ahn SS. The effectiveness of percutaneous transluminal angioplasty for the treatment of critical limb ischemia: A 10-year experience. *J Vasc Surg.* 41:423–435, 2005.

Lange S, Diehm C, Darius H, Haberl R, Allenberg JR, Pittrow D, Schuster A, von Stritzky B, Tepohl G, Trampisch HJ. High prevalence of peripheral arterial disease and low treatment rates in elderly primary care patients with diabetes. *Exp Clin Endocrinol Diabetes* 112:566–573, 2004.

Larsson J, Agardh CD, Apelqvist J, Stenstrom A. Long-term prognosis after healed amputation in patients with diabetes. *Clin Orthop Relat Res* 350:149–158, 1998.

Luscher TF, Creager MA, Beckman JA, Cosentino F. Diabetes and vascular disease: Pathophysiology, clinical consequences, and medical therapy: Part II. *Circulation* 108:1655–1661, 2003.

McLafferty RB, Dunnington GL, Mattos MA, Markwell SJ, Ramsey DE, Henretta JP, Karch LA, Hodgson KJ, Sumner DS. Factors affecting the diagnosis of peripheral vascular disease before vascular surgery referral. *J Vasc Surg* 31:870–879, 2000.

Menard JR, Smith HE, Riebe D, Braun CM, Blissmer B, Patterson RB. Long-term results of peripheral arterial disease rehabilitation. *J Vasc Surg* 39:1186–1192, 2004.

Morris AD, McAlpine R, Steinke D, Boyle DI, Ebrahim AR, Vasudev N, Stewart CP, Jung RT, Leese GP, MacDonald TM, Newton RW. Diabetes and lower-limb amputations in the community: A retrospective cohort study. *Diabetes Care* 21(5):738–743, 1998.

Moulik PK, Mtonga R, Gill GV. Amputation and mortality in new-onset diabetic foot ulcers stratified by etiology. *Diabetes Care* 26(2):491–494, 2003.

Muller IS, de Grauw WJ, van Gerwen WH, Bartelink ML, van Den Hoogen HJ, Rutten GE. Foot ulceration and lower limb amputation in type 2 diabetic patients in Dutch primary health care. *Diabetes Care* 25:570–574, 2002.

Nehler MR, Coll JR, Hiatt WR, Regensteiner JG, Schnickel GT, Klenke WA, Strecker PK, Anderson MW, Jones DN, Whitehill TA, Moskowitz S, Krupski WC. Functional outcome in a contemporary series of major lower extremity amputations. *J Vasc Surg* 38:7–14, 2003.

Ragnarson Tennvall G, Apelqvist J. Health-related quality of life in patients with diabetes mellitus and foot ulcers. *J Diabetes Complications* 14:235–241, 2000.

Skrha J, Ambos A. Can the atherosclerosis prevention targets be achieved in type 2 diabetes? *Diabetes Res Clin Prac* 68S1:S48–S51, 2005.

Tentolouris N, Al-Sabbagh S, Walker MG, Boulton AJ, Jude EB. Mortality in diabetic and nondiabetic patients after amputations performed from 1990 to 1995. *Diabetes Care* 27(7):1598–1604, 2004.

Townsend CM, Beauchamp RD, Evers BM, Mattox KL, Eds. *Sabiston Textbook of Surgery: The Biological Basis of Modern Surgical Practice*, 17th ed. Philadelphia: W.B. Saunders Company, 2004.

Suggested Reading

CAPRIE Steering Committee. A randomised, blinded trial of clopidogrel versus aspirin in patients at risk of ischaemic events (CAPRIE). *Lancet* 348:1329–1339, 1996.

Creager MA, Luscher TF, Cosentino F, Beckman JA. Diabetes and vascular disease: Pathophysiology, clinical consequences, and medical therapy: Part I. *Circulation* 108:1527–1532, 2003.

Dawson DL, Cutler BS, Hiatt WR, Hoboson RW, Martin JD, Bortey EB, Forbes WP, Strandness DE. A comparison of cilostazol and pentoxifylline for treating intermittent claudication. *Am J Med* 109:523–530, 2000.

Goshima KR, Mills JL Sr, Hughes JD. A new look at outcomes after infrainguinal bypass surgery: Traditional reporting standards underestimate the expenditure of effort required to attain limb salvage. *J Vasc Surg* 39(2):330–335, 2004.

Hirsch AT, Criqui MH, Treat-Jacobson D, Regensteiner JG, Creager MA, Olin JW, Krook SH, Hunninghake DB, Comerota AJ, Walsh ME, McDermott MM, Hiatt WR. Peripheral arterial disease: Detection, awareness, and treatment in primary care. *JAMA* 286(11):1317–1324, 2001.

Kalbaugh CA, Taylor SM, Cull DL, Blackhurst DW, Gray BH, Langan EM 3rd, Dellinger MB, McClary GE Jr, Jackson MR, Carsten CG 3rd, Snyder BA, York JW, Youkey JR. Invasive treatment of chronic limb ischemia according to the Lower Extremity Grading System (LEGS) Score: A 6-month report. *J Vasc Surg* 39:1268–1276, 2004.

Larsson J, Agardh CD, Apelqvist J, Stenstrom A. Long-term prognosis after healed amputation in patients with diabetes. *Clin Orthop Relat Res* 350:149–158, 1998.

2

Prevention and Healing of the Neuropathic Foot Ulceration

Stephanie A. Slayton, PT, DPT, CWS

Introduction

Diabetic foot ulcerations are a chronic wound type (Fig. 1). A wound that is deemed chronic is one that has failed to proceed through an orderly and timely process to produce anatomic and functional integrity, or proceeds through the repair process without establishing a sustained anatomic and functional result (Hess and Trent 2004). Tissue stresses common to the diabetic patient that cause delayed wound healing are compromised vascular supply, infection, and hyperkeratotic callus formation at the ulcer edge. Other factors that need to be controlled in order to allow wound healing are systemic and include hyperglycemia, oxygenation of tissue, and nutritional status. Patients with previous ulcerations are at increased risk for tissue breakdown because scar tissue is only 80% as strong as the original tissue. Within five years of developing a plantar ulcer, the cumulative recurrence rate of ulceration is estimated to be 70%, and the amputation rate is estimated to be, 12% (Horswell et al. 2003).

Wound healing requires an interdisciplinary approach (Table 1). All the members of the health care team must work together closely and treat the whole patient to optimize outcomes. The most important member of the team is the patient. Without his or her willingness to participate in the plan, healing is not possible. Many treatment options are available—some old, some new, but all aim to

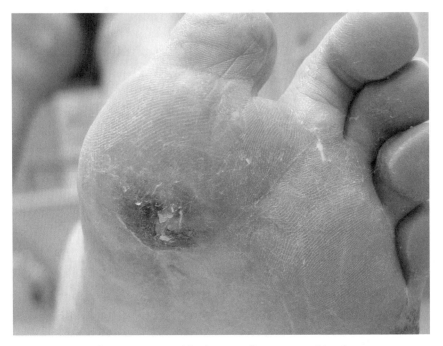

Figure 1 Neuropathic ulcer over first metatarsal head.

restore tissue integrity and prevent further ulcerations. A variety of health care professionals may utilize these treatments to promote healing.

Lower Extremity/Foot Assessment

Prevention/Patient Education

It has been estimated that 80% of diabetic ulcers are preventable (Reiber et al. 1999). Patient and family education is the most important aspect in the prevention

Table 1 Disciplines Providing Care

Physician
Nurse Practitioner
Podiatrist
Orthotist/Prosthetist
Nutritionist
Diabetes Specialist
Pharmacist
Physical Therapist
Occupational Therapist

and healing of diabetic foot ulcerations. Patients play the primary role in prevention and healing as they are the ones making decisions about their day-to-day activities. The importance of daily monitoring of glucose control, diet, and exercise should be stressed to the patient. Patients and their families should be taught to perform daily skin checks of the patients' lower extremities and instructed to avoid soaking their feet in warm water.

Examination of the Lower Extremity

A thorough examination of both lower extremities should be made, from the proximal leg to the distal aspect of the foot. Notation should be made of any bony deformities, hair growth patterns, temperature, and callus formation. This examination can give insight into any vascular compromise and increased plantar pressures. Note the location of any old scarring. Examine the heels for fissures, and between the toes for cracks and macerations (Fig. 2). Toenails should be

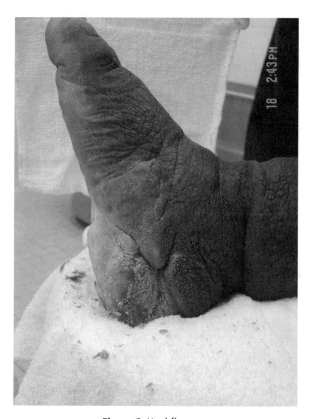

Figure 2 Heel fissures.

assessed for length, color, thickness, odor, and any complaints of pain. Note any pigment changes in the skin and the skin texture, such as anhydrosis and tinea (fungal infection).

An examination of the patient's shoes should also be made, noting the shoe type and wear patterns. This will assist with assessment for any abnormal gait pattern and will give you insight as to potential causes of ulceration from ill-fitting shoes. Diabetic patients should be referred to a qualified health care professional for custom molded diabetic shoes at least once a year. If a patient has a foot deformity, shoes need to be customized for them to reduce the plantar pressures, and the patient should be referred to a health care professional who is able to do so (e.g., certified pedorthist, certified prosthetist, or certified orthotist).

Gait Analysis and Balance Assessment

Gait and balance disturbances are due to muscle imbalances and alterations in joint range of motion. The most commonly observed gait abnormality is a foot flat pattern, with a loss of a heel strike. This gait abnormality produces increased loading time at the metatarsal heads. As patients begin to feel unsteady on their feet due to decreased sensation and proprioception they adapt a wider base of support to increase their stability.

Wound Assessment

Foot ulceration and infections are now the most common diabetes-related cause of hospitalization in the United States (Lipsky 1999). Wound location(s) should be noted, marked, and numbered on a body diagram to aid in consistent documentation. Common locations for diabetic neuropathic foot ulcerations are on the plantar aspect of the foot, under the metatarsal heads, and under the heel (Fig. 3). Documentation of wounds should include the use of anatomical terms for consistency of communication between health care professionals.

Wound Description

Neuropathic ulcers appear with a beefy red base and are usually surrounded by hyperkeratotic tissue, resembling a punched out lesion (Shapero et al. 2002). Description of the wound should include color and texture of the wound base, amount and consistency of wound exudate, and any odor. Description of the

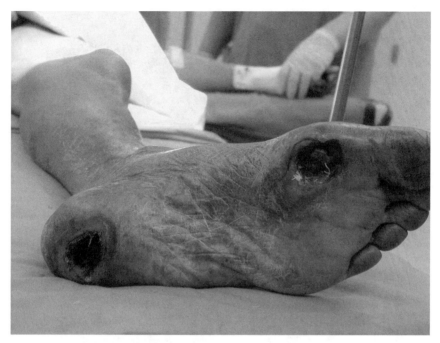

Figure 3 Ulcerations at heel and first metatarsal head. (Courtesy of Carolyn Horne, RN, CNS, East Carolina University Vascular Surgery Department)

wound base should include tissue type (eschar, fibrinous slough, granulation, re-epithelialization) and if any anatomic structure is present (bone, tendon, ligaments, vessels, nerves). If the wound extends down to bone, the patient should be referred to a physician for further testing to rule out osteomyelitis. Black eschar represents dried out tissue that tends to be firm. Fibrinous tissue may be firm or sloughy (stringy), and is typically yellow in color. Slough can be any number of colors based on the infectious organism that is present: white, yellow, blue-green, gray, brown, or black. The presence of necrotic tissue within the wound will impair the healing processes by stimulating inflammation and delaying granulation and epithelialization (Zacur and Kirsner 2002). Granulation tissue is red-pink in color, firm, moist, and appears to have small bumps. Re-epithelialization tissue forms at and advances from the edges of the wound or around epidermal accessories such as hair follicles, and tends to be pink-purple in color. Signs of infection should be noted which include purulence, inflammation, erythema/cellulitis, and tracking/tunneling/undermining. Figure 4 shows an example of hyperkeratosis in a neuropathic foot ulcer.

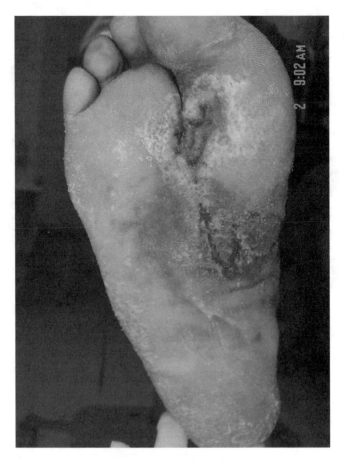

Figure 4 Hyperkeratosis.

Periwound Assessment

Diabetic neuropathic foot ulceration wound margins tend to be even with a deep wound bed. Periwound assessment should examine for callus formation, maceration, edema, or erythema. Callus (hyperkeratosis) formation can lead to increased plantar pressures. Calluses need to be removed and observed for reformation. It is generally believed that the presence of plantar callus is strongly associated with a high risk of ulceration (Spencer 2004). If callus continues to form, despite debridement, off-loading of the extremity with the orthotic or shoe is not adequate. Maceration of the periwound tissue occurs when exudate is not adequately controlled. Maceration can lead to further breakdown of the tissue and enlargement of the wound (Figs. 5 and 6).

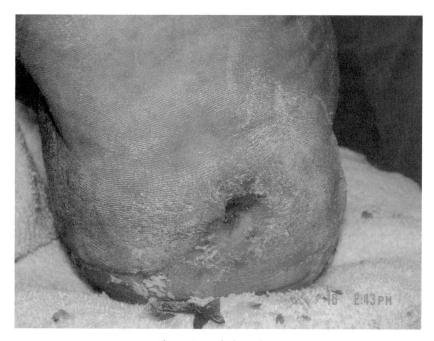

Figure 5 Heel ulceration.

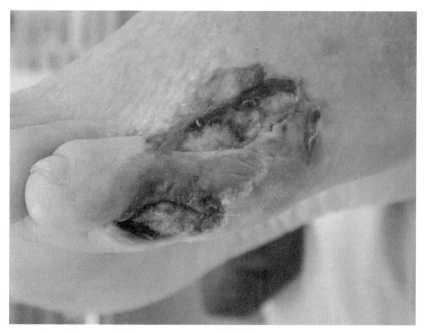

Figure 6 Ischemia of fifth digit. (Courtesy of Carolyn Horne, RN, CNS, East Carolina University Vascular Surgery Department)

Exudate

Due to their inflammatory state, chronic wounds often produce copious amounts of exudate (Enoch and Harding 2003). Debriding and cleaning the wound is the first step in managing excessive exudate, but long-term management requires use of modern dressings (Enoch and Harding 2003). Exudate can be detrimental to the wound (Sibbald et al. 2000).

Exudate is usually described by quantity (scant, moderate, copious), characteristics (serous, sanguinous, purulent, or a combination), and any odor. Diabetic foot ulcerations tend to have low to moderate amounts of drainage unless infected. Increasing amounts of exudate should alert a clinician of underlying problems.

Odor

Upon removal of the dressing, an odor will be present. This is due to the saturation and warming of the dressing with exudate. Prior to the assessment, if a wound odor is present or absent, a cleansing of the wound must occur. If wound odor is present, a description of the odor should be documented.

Classification

Based on lower extremity (LE) assessment and wound evaluation, a determination of wound etiology can be made. Neuropathic wounds are commonly classified using one of the two commonly used systems: the Wagner Ulcer Classification and The University of Texas Health Science Center Diabetic Wound Classification system. Classification systems are useful to help standardize documentation and make communication between clinicians easier.

The Wagner Diabetic Foot Ulceration Classification system was developed in 1981 as a way for health care providers to communicate more effectively with one another (Wagner 1981). It is used to record the presence of depth and infection or necrosis in a wound (Table 2). Ulcer grading is useful for prognosis and selection of treatment interventions. A downfall of this system is that it does not provide for the description of concomitant conditions (Armstrong and Peters 2001).

In an attempt to include the concomitant conditions that can affect wound healing, the University of Texas Health Science Center Diabetic Wound Classification system was established (Table 3) (Armstrong, Lavery, and Harkless 1998; Lavery, Armstrong, and Harkless 1996). This system is based on assessing the wound as follows: 1) its depth and 2) whether it is infected, ischemic, or both (Armstrong and Peters 2001). This system takes into account known risk factors that influence the prognosis of the wound.

Table 2 Wagner Diabetic Foot Ulceration Classification

Grade 0	Pre-ulcerative lesions; healed ulcers; bony deformity present
Grade 1	Superficial ulcer without subcutaneous involvement
Grade 2	Penetration through subcutaneous tissue; may expose bone, tendon, ligament, or joint capsule
Grade 3	Osteitis, abscess, or osteomyelitis
Grade 4	Gangrene of a digit
Grade 5	Gangrene of foot requiring disarticulation

Table 3 University of Texas Health Science Center Diabetic Wound Classification System (Armstrong, Lavery, and Harkless 1998; Lavery, Armstrong, and Harkless 1996)

	GRADE/DEPTH				
	0	**I**	**II**	**III**	**S**
A	Pre- or post-ulcerative lesion completely epithelialized	Superficial wound not involving tendon, capsule, or bone	Wound penetrating to tendon or capsule	Wound penetrating to bone or joint	**T**
B	Pre- or post-ulcerative lesion completely epithelialized with infection	Superficial wound not involving tendon, capsule, or bone with infection	Wound penetrating to tendon or capsule with infection	Wound penetrating to bone or joint with infection	**A**
C	Pre- or post-ulcerative lesion completely epithelialized with ischemia	Superficial wound not involving tendon, capsule, or bone with ischemia	Wound penetrating to tendon or capsule with ischemia	Wound penetrating to bone or joint with ischemia	**G**
D	Pre- or post-ulcerative lesion completely epithelialized with infection & ischemia	Superficial wound not involving tendon, capsule, or bone with infection & ischemia	Wound penetrating to tendon or capsule with infection and ischemia	Wound penetrating to bone or joint with infection and ischemia	**E**

Laboratory Assessments

Blood Glucose

Capillary plasma glucose levels should range from 90–130 mg/dl, according to the ADA (2005). Hyperglycemia affects protein synthesis, white cell function, oxygen transportation and utilization, and growth factor availability (Falanga 2002). The U.K. Prospective Diabetes Study showed that improved glycemic control is associated with sustained decreased rates of retinopathy, nephropathy, and neuropathy (ADA 2005).

Hemoglobin A1C

Hemoglobin A1C (HbA1C) is an aggregate of the patient's glucose level over a 90-day period, the lifespan of a red blood cell. Normal A1C is 4%–6.0%. The goal for a diabetic patient is less than 7% according to the ADA (2005). ADA recommends performance of the A1C test at least twice a year in patients who are meeting their treatment goals, and quarterly in those who are not (ADA 2005). Chronically elevated glucose levels will be represented by a higher HbA1C, which leads to microvascular damage, inhibits oxygen and nutrition perfusion, and hampers wound healing (Hess and Trent 2004).

Albumin/Pre-Albumin

Another important lab result is the patient's albumin and prealbumin levels, which are a measure of serum protein levels. A patient's normal albumin level is 3.5–5.4 g/100 mL, and prealbumin is 23–43 mg/100 mL. As a patient's blood glucose level rises the body believes it is in a catabolic state and begins to break down protein the body has stored. This places a patient at increased risk for skin breakdown, and makes it very difficult to heal an already present wound.

Total Lymphocyte Count (TLC)

TLC can give insight to the clinician if an infection is present without the classic clinical signs and symptoms. Normal TLC is >2000/μL.

Wound Healing in the Diabetic Patient

Even with the most advanced technologies, wound healing in the diabetic population is impossible without control of their blood glucose. Management is determined by the severity and duration of ulceration, the vascularity, and the presence or absence of infection (Frykberg 2002). Unless the previously named items are addressed, wound care is likely to fail no matter what modality or dressing choices are used.

Wound bed preparation can be defined as the global management of the wound to accelerate endogenous healing or to facilitate the effectiveness of other therapeutic measures (Falanga 2002). Chronic wounds have "necrotic burden," consisting of both necrotic tissue and exudate (Falanga 2002). An important aspect of wound bed preparation is the recognition that chronic wounds have the underlying pathogenic abnormalities that cause necrotic tissue accumulation (Enoch and Harding 2003).

Off-Loading of the Lower Extremity

Because pressure, shear, and repetitive injury are a few of the causative factors behind ulceration in the diabetic patient, they must be reduced and removed in order to heal already ulcerated tissue and to prevent future ulcerations. Selection of the appropriate method of off-loading foot ulcerations is often based on many factors including the size and severity of the wound, duration of ulceration, patient's age, clinician's experience and judgment, patient preference, cost, and time (Birke et al. 2004).

Total contact casting (TCC) has been shown to be the gold standard in reducing and redistributing plantar pressures. TCC reduces plantar pressures at the site of ulceration by 84%–92% (Armstrong et al. 2005). The cast is effective because it reduces pressure over the ulcer area, imposes continuous offloading, reduces edema, and limits patient activity (Birke et al. 2004). A limiting factor with TCC is that it negates the ability to view the wound daily (Shapero et al. 2002). Therefore, TCC is contraindicated for diabetic foot ulcerations with soft tissue infections or osteomyelitis (Shapero et al. 2002; see Yamada, Chapter 3, page 41).

Useful devices to assist in off-loading include the standard and rolling walker, crutches, canes, and wheelchair. The disadvantage of a cane is that the limb cannot be completely off-loaded as it can with the other assistive devices. Wheelchairs are beneficial in that both lower extremities can be off-loaded at the same time. Compliance with the use of these devices is patient-driven. Patient education is the key to making the patient understand the role of pressure in ulceration development and healing.

Debridement

Necrotic tissue contains dead cells and debris that changes color from red to brown or black/purple as it becomes more dehydrated, and finally forms a black, dry, thick, and leathery structure known as eschar (Enoch and Harding 2003). During the early debridement stage, a wound may actually increase in size before it contracts (Sibbald et al. 2000). Debridement involves the removal of dead, devitalized, or contaminated tissue, and any foreign material from a wound. Aggressive debridement of the wound and periwound is of utmost importance to prepare the wound bed for healing.

Removal of devitalized tissue can be achieved through many forms of debridement. An ideal wound debriding agent is one that is selective to nonviable tissue. Mechanical debridement includes pulsed irrigation with suction and whirlpool for cleansing. Soaking of ulcers is controversial and should be avoided because the neuropathic patient can easily be scaled by hot water (Frykberg 2002). Haynes et al. compared the effects of pulsed lavage and whirlpool on the rate of formation of granulation tissue in 13 subjects with a variety of chronic wounds (Haynes 1994). The rate of granulation tissue formation for patients receiving pulsed lavage (12.2% per week) was greater than the granulation rate of patients receiving whirlpool (4.8% per week; Haynes 1994).

Sharp debridement is the fastest form of debridement. Studies by Steed et al. confirmed that patients with diabetic neuropathic foot ulcers who underwent regular sharp debridement did better than those whose ulcers had less debridement (Steed 1996). Sharp debridement is also an effective way to remove callus formation and reduce periwound pressure.

Advanced Debridement Techniques

MIST Therapy System (Celleration Inc., Eden Prairie, Minn.)

The MIST therapy system is a low-frequency (40 KHz), noncontact ultrasound device FDA cleared for the cleansing and debridement of wounds. Treatment duration is approximately five minutes, but can vary depending on size of the wound.

Ultrasonic Assisted Wound Treatment (SÖRING GmbH–Sonoca UAW 180)

The Sonoca UAW 180 (SÖRING GmbH) is a low-frequency (25 kHz), contact ultrasound device. The device is effective in the gentle but fast debridement of wounds with decreased pain when compared to surgical debridement. Indications for use include debridement of infected, necrotic, and ischemic wounds. Recommendations for clinical use include chronic diabetic foot ulcers, arterial ulcers, and venous ulcers.

Wound Healing Modalities

Monochromatic Infrared Therapy (MIRE)

Infrared is a radiating energy or waveform. Infrared passes through human tissues until it is absorbed or diffuses. The therapeutic wavelength range is 590 nm–1000 nm for tissue repair. The nonthermal delivery of infrared is believed to be beneficial for encouraging progression through the inflammatory phase and enhancing the proliferation phase, including angiogenesis, and remodeling.

Anodyne® (Anodyne Therapy, LLC, Tampa, FL) MIRE therapy is a light emitting diode (LED) with 59 monochromatic (890 nm) near-infrared emitters. The LED pads conform to and maintain contact with the treatment area with the assistance of a strap and are placed both on the wound and on the periwound skin. This treatment modality was approved by the FDA in 1994 to increase circulation, decrease inflammation, reduce edema, and decrease pain. Tables 4 and 5 show the recommended treatment protocols for neuropathy and wound healing using Anodyne Therapy.

Ultraviolet–C

Ultraviolet light treatment is a topical noncontact treatment that has been used for wound healing for years. The antimicrobial effects of light have been demonstrated

Table 4 Recommended Treatment Protocol for Neuropathy (Anodyne)

Once-daily use for 90 days
30–40 Minutes/limb
4 Therapy pads/limb
6–8 Bars of intensity (10 bars = maximum intensity)
After 90 days, decrease frequency to no less than 1-2x/week

Table 5 Recommended Treatment Protocol for Wound Healing (Anodyne)

Treat directly over wound for best results, cover wound with film dressing
Treat over skin to treat undermined areas
Inpatient—treat daily
Home health—at each dressing change
Minimum 3x/week
30 Minutes/treatment
6–8 Bars of intensity (10 bars = maximum)

as far back as 1877 in an experiment performed by Downed and Blunt (Licht 1967).

Current recommendations for treating infected wounds suggest use of a cold quartz lamp, 1 inch from the wound surface for 72–180 seconds. It has been found that UVC will not penetrate through a thin film dressing (Sullivan et al. 1999). Current recommendations are to remove all dressings prior to treatment with UVC lamp.

Ultrasound

Clinical (nonthermal) therapy is primarily used in wound healing for the debridement of dermal ulcerations. Ultrasound therapy requires a medium between the ultrasound head and the skin. Gels and lotions can be used on areas where good contact can be made, but for irregular surfaces (such as the ankle or toes), water in a plastic bucket may be the best medium.

Ultrasound has been shown to be most effective when started during the inflammatory phase, although benefits can be seen by using ultrasound in all phases of healing.

Electrical Stimulation

Multiple randomized controlled trials and clinical trials have shown that electrical stimulation in conjunction with standard wound care practices accelerates the healing rate of chronic wounds as compared to standard wound care alone. Electrical stimulation is FDA-approved for wound healing in a chronic wound that has failed standard treatment (Table 6).

Table 6 Physiological Responses with E-Stim

Increased blood flow
Increased oxygenation
Increased cell migration (neutrophils, macrophages, lymphocytes, fibroblasts)
Increased collagen production
Increased growth factor production
Bacteriostatic
Activation of fibroblasts (increase DNA, collagen synthesis, increase growth
    factor receptor sites)

Table 7 Beneficial Effects of HBO in Wound Healing (Broussard 2004)

Decreased local tissue edema
Improved cellular energy metabolism
Improved local tissue oxygenation
Improved leukocyte-killing ability
Increased effectiveness of antibiotics
Enhanced uptake of platelet-derived growth factor-BB
Promotion of collagen deposition
Promotion of neoangiogenesis
Enhanced epithelial migration

Hyperbaric Oxygen Therapy

Centers for Medicare and Medicaid Services approved reimbursement for the adjunctive use of hyperbaric oxygenation (HBO) in August of 2003, for the use in patients with diabetes mellitus and a Wagner Grade III wound of the lower extremity resulting from diabetes, which has not responded to standard wound care treatment (Centers for Medicare and Medicaid Service 2006). HBO is the administration of 100% oxygen at greater than one atmosphere pressure absolute (ATA). Topical application of oxygen to a wound is not HBO. HBO therapy is administered usually once daily for wound care (Table 7). See Chapter 5 for a detailed discussion on HBO.

Wound Dressings

The key to good wound healing is to keep the wound clean, free of devitalized tissue, and to keep it moist. A moist wound surface prevents desiccation and cell death, and enhances epithelial migration. Dressings are chosen based on assessment of the wound and periwound, and conformability of the dressing.

Standard Dressings

Standard dressings come in many forms, from the basic gauze to a more advanced calcium alginate and foam. Wet to dry gauze dressings are a thing of the past, as newer dressings which better promote moist wound healing have come into favor. Standard dressings should be considered when choosing a dressing, and continual clinical assessment will allow for appropriate dressings to be used at the appropriate time in the healing process.

Subatmospheric Therapy

Theory

Negative pressure wound therapy (NPWT) is used for a multitude of wound types, including diabetic foot ulcerations. Subatmospheric pressure has been proposed to alter the wound environment by reducing bacterial load and chronic interstitial wound exudate, increasing vascularity and cytokine expression, and physically contracting wound margins (Claxton, Armstrong, and Boulton 2002). In theory, applied negative pressure will stimulate development of granulation tissue in a previously nonhealing wound leading to epithelialization (Tucson Expert Consensus Conference 2004).

KCI—Wound Vacuum Assisted Closure (V.A.C.)® (*KCI USA, San Antonio, TX*)

This modality entails placing sterile foam cut to the size of the wound into the wound bed. A dime-sized hole is cut in the center of the film and tubing is placed that is then attached to the adjustable vacuum source, which can provide negative pressure therapy continuously or intermittently. V.A.C.® Instill™, which combines the benefits of negative pressure wound therapy with an automated delivery of topical solutions to the wound site is also available. See Chapter 6 for a detailed discussion of V.A.C.

Advanced Dressings

Silver

All products are not created equal. The amount of silver available in different dressings and creams is variable and often uncontrolled. The biocidal properties of silver ions were first investigated in 1869 (Thomas and McCubbin 2003). Many silver-containing dressings are available. Application of a silver product should be based on wound environment and the bacterial load of the wound.

Cadexomer Iodine (*Health Point, Inc., Fort Worth, TX*)

Iodosorb® gel and Iodoflex™ pads are produced by HealthPoint. Both products are composed of cadexomer iodine that is slowly released into the wound fluid. Application is directly to the wound bed, ensuring complete contact, and then covered with a dressing. The dressing is left in place for up to three days or until the dressing turns from a brown to yellowish color.

Bioengineered Skin Substitutes

This therapy is also known as human skin equivalent tissue and offers the possibility of creating physiologically compatible skin. The principal goal behind use of skin substitutes is to prevent infection and to allow the wound to heal by normal processes.

Apligraf (Organogenesis, Canton, MA, and Novartis Pharmaceuticals, East Hanover, NJ) is derived from fibroblasts of neonatal foreskins. The graft is bilayered consisting of an epidermis and dermis. Apligraf has FDA approval for venous insufficiency ulcers and diabetic foot ulcerations.

Dermagraft (Advanced Tissue Sciences/Smith & Nephew Inc., La Jolla, CA and Largo, FL) is a dissolvable mesh framework of bovine collagen containing cultured neonatal fibroblasts. Dermagraft is designed to replace the dermis and provide essential stimulatory growth factors (Braddock, Campbell, Zuder 1999). This product is approved by the FDA for full-thickness diabetic foot ulcers.

Growth Factors

Platelet-Derived Growth Factor (PDGF)

Genetically engineered platelet-derived growth factor becaplermin (Regranex; Johnson and Johnson Wound Management, A Division of ETHICON, Inc.) is FDA approved on diabetic foot ulcerations. Application of PDGF is once daily with twice a day dressing changes. The ointment should be left in place for 12 hours. For the growth factor to be effective the diabetic foot ulcer needs to be free of necrotic tissue prior to application and have a good vascular supply.

Conclusion

This chapter is meant to be an overview of the importance of neuropathic wound assessment, and of the variety of modalities and dressings available for treatment. To heal a neuropathic ulcer effectively, all components of the patient need to be addressed. This holistic approach to patient care requires a multidisciplinary approach.

Patients being treated with any of the previously mentioned procedures should be under the direct care of a licensed health care provider who is trained in the application of the modality. Wound care clinicians are educated in identifying the ever-changing wound environment and determining the best intervention and care for the wound. For health care professionals who are involved in the treatment of wounds, frequent education through journals and continuing education courses is of utmost importance.

References

American Diabetes Association. Standards of medical care in diabetes. *Diabetes Care* 28 (Supp 1):S4–S20, 2005.

Anodyne Therapy, LLC. www.anodynetherapy.com January 2006.

Armstrong DG, Peters EJG. Classification of wounds of the diabetic foot. *Curr Diabetes Rep* 1:233–238, 2001.

Armstrong DG, Lavery LA, Harkless LB. Validation of a diabetic wound classification system. *Diabetes Care* 21:855–858, 1998.

Armstrong DG, Lavery LA, Wu S, Boulton AJ. Evaluation of removable and irremovable cast walkers in the healing of diabetic foot wounds: A randomized controlled trial. *Diabetes Care* 28(3):551–554, 2005.

Birke J, Lewis K, Penton A, Pittman D, Tucker A, Durand C. The effectiveness of a modified wedge shoe in reducing pressure at the area of previous great toe ulceration in Individuals with diabetes mellitus. *Wounds* 16(4):109–114, 2004.

Braddock M, Campbell CJ, Zuder D. Current therapies for wound healing: Electrical stimulation, biological therapeutics, and the potential for gene therapy. *Int J Dermatol* 38:808–817, 1999.

Broussard CL. Hyperbaric oxygenation and wound healing. *J Vascular Nursing* 22:42–48, 2004.

Centers for Medicare and Medicaid Services. www.cms.hhs.gov/, January 2006.

Claxton MJ, Armstrong DG, Boulton AJM. Healing the diabetic wound and keeping it healed: Modalities for the early 21st century. *Curr Diabetes Rep* 2:510–518, 2002.

Enoch S, Harding K. Wound bed preparation: The science behind the removal of barriers to healing. *Wounds* 15:213–229, 2003.

Falanga V. Wound bed preparation and the role of enzymes: A case for multiple Actions of therapeutic agents. *Wounds* 14:47–57, 2002.

Frykberg RG. Diabetic foot ulcers: Pathogenesis and management. *Am Fam Physicians* 66: 1645–1661, 2002.

Haynes LJ, Brown MH, Handley BC, et al. Comparison of Pulsavac and sterile whirlpool regarding the promotion of tissue granulation [abstract]. *Phys Ther* 74(suppl):S4, 1994.

Hess CT, Trent JT. Incorporating laboratory values in chronic wound management. *Adv Skin Wound Care* 17:378–386, 2004.

Horswell RL, Birke JA, Patout CA Jr. A staged management diabetes foot program versus standard care: A 1-year cost and utilization comparison in a state public hospital system. *Arch Phys Med Rehabil* 84:1743–1746, 2003.

Lavery LA, Armstrong DG, Harkless LB. Classification of diabetic foot wounds. *J Foot Ankle Surg* 35:528–531, 1996.

Licht S. *Therapeutic Electricity and Ultraviolet Radiation.* Baltimore, MD: Waverly Press, Inc. 1967.

Lipsky BA. A current approach to diabetic foot infections. *Curr Infect Dis Rep* 1:253–259, 1999.

Reiber GE, Vileikyte L, Boyko EJ, del Aguila M, Smith DG, Lavery LA, Boulton AJ. Causal pathways for incident lower-extremity ulcers in patients with diabetes from two settings. *Diabetes Care* 22(1):157–161, 1999.

Shapero C et al. A review of off-loading techniques for the treatment of diabetic plantar neuropathic ulcerations. *Acute Care Perspect* 11:3–6, 2002.

Sibbald RG, Orsted H, Schultz GS, Coutts P, Keast D; International Wound Bed Preparation Advisory Board; Canadian Chronic Wound Advisory Board. Preparing the wound bed—Debridement, bacterial balance, and moisture balance. *Ostomy Wound Manage* 46: 14–35, 2000.

Steed DL, Donohoe D, Webster MW, Lindsley L. Effect of extensive debridement and treatment on healing of diabetic foot ulcers. *J Am Coll Surg* 183:60–63, 1996.

Spencer S. Pressure relieving interventions for preventing and treating diabetic foot ulcers (Cochrane Review). In *The Cochrane Library*, Issue 1, 2004. Chichester, UK: John Wiley & Sons, Ltd.

Thomas S, McCubbin P. A comparison of the antimicrobial effects of four silver-containing dressings on three organisms. *J Wound Care* 12:101–107, 2003.

Tucson Expert Consensus Conference. Guidelines regarding negative wound therapy (NPWT) in the diabetic foot. *Ostomy Wound Manage* 50(4 Suppl B):3S–27S, 2004.

Wagner F. The dysvascular foot: A system for diagnosis and treatment. *Foot Ankle* 2:63–122, 1981.

Zacur H, Kirsner RS. Debridement: Rationale and therapeutic options. *Wounds* 14(7 Suppl): 2E–7E, 2002.

Suggested Reading

Organogenesis www.apligraf.com January 2006.

SÖRING—Sonoca UAW 180. www.soering.de/ January 2006.

3

Partial Foot Amputations

Wesley N. Yamada, DPM

Introduction

Preservation of foot structure and function, and maintenance of skin integrity are key goals of preventative diabetic foot care. However, amputation is sometimes an inevitable result of gangrene/ischemia or overwhelming infection.

Amputation, at any level, alters the integrity of the foot and results in abnormal biomechanical stresses that are placed on the remaining structure. Deformity, transfer lesions, ulcerations, fracture, and Charcot osteoarthropathy are possible consequences.

Level of amputation is an important factor. Foot, or distal, amputations are preferable to more proximal leg amputation. These amputations require minimal or no prosthetic device to maintain a patient as an independent ambulator. There is also less risk of phantom limb pain. Patient factors to be considered include emotional impact of amputation, body self-image, and limited cardiopulmonary reserve. Proximal amputation increases metabolic demands during walking and decreases self-selected walking speed and stride length, negatively affecting patients' independence and quality of life. While amputation is the last resort when treating a diabetic patient, one must be prepared to deal with the consequences if it occurs.

Digital Amputation

Hallux or Big Toe Amputation

The hallux is the most important toe of the foot. It bears more body weight versus the lesser toes during the final phase of gait, and it stabilizes the medial column of the foot (the medial column is, in essence, the medial half of the foot, comprised of the 1st through 3rd toes, metatarsals, cuneiforms, and navicular). It also provides overall balance to the foot during the end of single limb stance, and allows a smooth transference of body weight from the lateral aspect of the foot to the medial during the final stages of gait.

If the hallux is lost due to amputation, an imbalance of the remaining muscles occurs that affects foot function, which can lead to deformity. Additionally, because there is no hallux to bear weight, these forces (pressure and stresses) are transferred proximally and laterally.

Imbalance of Muscle Contraction/Deformity

After amputation of the hallux, an imbalance is created in the remaining foot muscles: They fire excessively and prematurely in an attempt to stabilize the foot. This creates a pull on the lesser toes, which causes hammertoe deformities. This also causes extension at the metatarsal-phalangeal joint (MTPJ) and flexion at the proximal interphalangeal joint (PIPJ) of the remaining toes. The second toe is the most affected, eventually leading to a clawtoe deformity (flexion at both the proximal and distal interphalangeal joints [DIPJ], respectively).

The vectors of pull of the remaining muscles are also changed with hallux amputation. The pull is now from a more medial direction and a varus force is created on the lesser digits. This causes them to rotate laterally, which can create callus formation on the plantar/lateral aspect of the toe.

As hammertoe deformities progress, anterior displacement of the fat pad beneath the MTPJ occurs, leaving unprotected metatarsal heads vulnerable to callus formation and ulceration (Pulla and Kaminsky 1997).

When the toe moves into a hammered position, the distal pulp (tip) of the toe becomes the only weight-bearing surface for the involved digit. This creates a dorsal force during stance or gait. This pushes the already buckled proximal interphalangeal joint up into the top of the toe box, which can create a blister or callus. The toe box tries to resist this force and pushes the proximal aspect of the toe plantarly. This increase in force is continued to the plantar MTPJ, which may cause a blister or callus. The force from the toe box is also directed to the distal aspect of the toe, causing an increase of pressure or friction, leading to a distal tip blister/callus.

Transfer of Pressure: Transfer Lesion Formation

At heel contact, body weight is primarily centered over the lateral half of the foot; from midstance on the weight is transferred distally and medially. At push off, the weight is centered over the metatarsal heads (MTHs) and digits, primarily the 1st and 2nd MTHs.

Hallux amputation creates instability of the medial column, which will be discussed in the next section. This instability causes a late, lateral shift in body weight during the latter phase of gait. The 2nd MTPJ is commonly affected by this lateral shift in pressure. Because of the increased pressure, a transfer lesion (callus or ulceration) may develop.

The initial presentation of the transfer lesion is hyperkeratosis under the second MTH. A hyperkeratotic lesion increases the local pressure by 30%, and, if left untreated, will undergo pressure necrosis, leading to ulceration (Levin 1995). Frequent sites of callus formation occur on the ball of the foot and digits after hallux amputation, especially involving the 2nd through 3rd MTPJs (Quebedeaux, Lavery L, and Lavery D 1996). If the transfer of pressure is great enough, a fracture rather than a lesion may occur. This is usually seen at the neck of the metatarsal, but can occur anywhere along the shaft.

Although less common, weight is not transferred laterally and an increase in pressure develops beneath the 1st metatarsal head, leading to the development of hyperkeratotic lesions or ulceration (Poppen et al. 1981). Also, callus patterns occur on the plantar aspect of the contralateral hallux, most likely due to altered biomechanics resulting from compensatory gait patterns.

Medial Column Instability

The medial column is stabilized by the plantar aponeurosis and plantar intrinsic muscles that insert onto the hallux. These soft tissues help maintain the height of the medial longitudinal arch in an analogous fashion as a string maintains the arch of a bow. When these supporting tissues are lost, the medial column no longer has plantar reinforcement and is more prone to collapse beneath the weight of the body (Poppen et al. 1981).

The increased medial ground reactive force places abnormal stress at the metatarsal cuneiform joint(s), causing dorsal jamming of the joint, which may lead to dorsal exostosis formation or Charcot osteoarthropathy.

Clinical Manifestations

It is important to inform patients of possible complications of hallux amputation: hammertoe or clawtoe formation, Charcot osteoarthropathy, and flattening of the foot and widening of the arch.

Hammertoes are defined as the curling of the toe at the MTPJ (dorsally) and PIPJ (plantarly). In clawtoe deformity, the DIPJ is also curled plantarly. Hammering or clawing of all the lesser toes may occur but the second toe is especially affected, hammering or clawing within the first year after amputation (Fig. 1).

Because only the MTH and distal tip of the toe purchase the ground with these deformities, the following clinical manifestations may occur:

1. Blister or callus formation at the end of the toe, on the top knuckle of the toe (PIPJ), or on the bottom of the foot under the 2nd toe joint (MTPJ) (Fig. 2).
2. The clinical signs of Charcot osteoarthropathy are swelling and redness at the lesser toe joints. Charcot is an uncontrolled breakdown of bone and joint usually seen in a well-perfused, neuropathic foot. In hallux

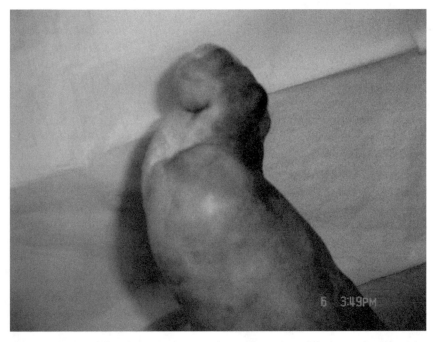

Figure 1 Clawtoe deformity. Note the extension at the MTPJ and flexion at the PIPJ and DIPJ.

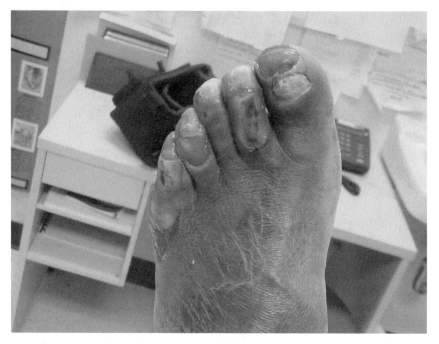

Figure 2 Ulcerations caused by neuropathy, digital deformity, and improperly fitted shoes.

amputation, Charcot can occur at the lesser MTPJs or, less commonly, at the medial midfoot (metatarsal-cuneiform joint[s]). This entity must be treated immediately by a clinician and all walking and standing on the foot should be stopped at once.

3. Flattening of the arch and widening of the foot is also a possible complication.

Treatment

Foot orthoses control flattening of the arch (also known as pronation). Most of the untoward sequelae following amputation are from medial column/foot instability. As the medial column collapses, the arch falls and pronatory forces at the subtalar joint are created. When the subtalar joint goes into a pronated position, it unlocks key joints in the foot that provide stability during gait. The structural integrity of the foot during all of stance is lost. Hammertoe deformities, flattening/widening of the foot, and jamming of the metatarsal-cuneiform joint are all caused by excessive pronation of the foot and can be attenuated with custom-made foot orthoses. Orthoses for diabetic patients should be made of materials that provide both flexibility and support. Orthoses made of only rigid materials (used for more functional control of the foot) should be avoided. Full-length top covers made of a combination of soft materials (for example, plastizote-1/poron combination) will provide cushioning as well as accommodation for callus formation under bony prominences.

Ankle-foot orthoses that control both internal rotation of the lower leg and subtalar joint eversion can also be used. Internal leg rotation and subtalar joint eversion are the key factors in the formation of pronatory forces in the foot, and if they are severe, a foot orthosis alone will not provide adequate control. Foot *and* leg motion must be restricted, especially in the coronal and transverse plane. Examples of such commercially available devices are the Arizona Ankle Brace® and the Richie Brace®.

Ortho-digital appliances (toe spacers) can be incorporated into the orthotic. Care must be exercised when using fixed ortho-digital appliances because they can cause irritation to the lesser digit next to the amputated hallux as well as to distal aspect of the residual foot. Close examination of the amputation site and adjacent areas must be performed by both patient and provider to prevent complications.

Extra-depth or custom-made shoes are also used. Depending on the degree and severity of the deformity, an extra-depth or custom shoe must be prescribed. Key factors in the proper selection of these shoes include ample room in the toe area to accommodate digital contractures or osseous prominences in the forefoot, soft upper materials, anatomical lasts to prevent toe crowding, and a strong heel counter to control the hind foot and maintain structural integrity of shoe.

Rocker bottom shoe modification will assist smooth roll over and a heel-toe gait. The modification distributes force over a greater area and advances stance more quickly and efficiently. Because body weight is more dispersed, pressure under areas such as the metatarsal heads is diminished. Padded hosiery, fitted properly with shoes, has also been shown to produce a significant reduction in both peak pressure and pressure over time (Veves et al. 1989). The decrease in pressure can help reduce the production of transfer lesions/ulcers.

Surgical correction of digital deformities may be required. Surgical fusion of the PIPJ and flexor tendon releases at the DIPJ and extensor tendon recession with lengthening at the MTPJ will surgically straighten the toe and improve function. The straightened alignment will help prevent callus/ulcer formation on the toe and beneath the affected metatarsal head.

For patients with Charcot, immediate nonweightbearing with immobilization until edema resolution, followed by total contact casting for 4–8 weeks, is the treatment.

The Charcot Resistant Orthotic Walker (CROW), also known as the total contact ankle foot orthosis (AFO) is a custom-formed lightweight "clam-shell" plastic device incorporating a custom foot orthosis. This should be used as a transitional device after short leg or total contact casting.

Arizona Ankle Brace® or Richie Brace® are both used when appropriate. Other modalities include electrical bone stimulation, bisphosphonates, and surgical fusion of affected joints (only after the quiescent or remodeling phases).

Lesser Toes

Amputation of the 2nd through 4th digits results in a loss of physiologic buttresses to adjacent toes. Often there will be drifting of the adjacent toes toward the void left by amputation. This occurs because of shoe pressure and altered firing of muscle groups to compensate for the lost digit as described in the previous section on hallux amputation.

Loss of the 5th digit presents the least deformity of the remaining digits after surgery. Because the anatomic pull of the tendons to the toes is toward a medial direction, the 1st through 4th digits rarely drift laterally with 5th toe loss. Fifth ray stability is altered, however, and a transfer lesion may develop under the 4th metatarsal head.

Partial Amputations of Lesser Toes

Amputation at the PIPJ level is difficult to manage because of the mechanical imbalances that are created through this joint. Because of the functional insertion of the extensor apparatus into the base of the proximal phalanx, the extensor tendons gain a mechanical advantage at this level, and the digit frequently develops an extension deformity with resultant ulcerations from rubbing on the shoe (Stuck et al. 1995).

Multiple Amputations of Toes

When three or more digits are amputated, the resultant deformation of the remaining toes renders them functionless. They become at risk for trauma, ulceration, and infection because the toes are more prone to getting "stubbed" or "caught" on bedding or hosiery. Fitting shoes becomes a difficult task and should never be undertaken without the supervision of a foot care provider.

Clinical Manifestations

Clinical manifestations include bunion formation, Tailor's bunion formation, hammertoe formation of the remaining toes, and flattening of the arch and widening of the foot.

1. Bunion formation is seen if the 2nd (primarily) and/or 3rd toes are amputated. The hallux begins to drift toward the space created by the amputated digit. As the deformity progresses, a prominent medial 1st MTPJ develops.
2. Tailor's bunion formation is the prominence of the 5th MTPJ (laterally) created by the loss of the 4th and/or 3rd toe(s).
3. Hammertoe (curling) formation of the remaining toes occurs with blister or callus formation at the distal pulp of the toe, DIPJ, or beneath the MTPJs. Varus rotation (twisting of the toes in the frontal plane so that the lateral surface of the toe becomes the weight-bearing surface) of the toes can also occur. Because the lateral surface is not endowed with as much fat padding as the plantar surface, callus and ulceration formation occurs more readily.
4. Flattening of the arch and widening of the foot is possible, but it is not as prevalent as with hallux amputation unless multiple toes are amputated.

Treatment

There are several different treatments when multiple amputations of toes are required:

1. Orthoses control flattening of the arch (see Hallux Amputation Treatment section).
2. An ortho-digital appliance fabricated from any soft, compliant material such as moldable podiatric compound, Plastizote 1, poron, or foam can prevent digital drift (Fig. 3). If the spacer is too bulky, however, it may cause irritation due to pressure from the inside of the shoe (Moore 1997). This is especially important in preventing bunion or Tailor's bunion formation.
3. Extra-depth or custom-made shoes, with a rocker bottom modification, are also effective options (see Hallux Amputation Treatment section).
4. Padded hosiery can also be effective as a treatment option (see Hallux Amputation Treatment section).
5. Surgical correction of digital deformities may also be necessary. Surgical fusion of the remaining toes should be performed only if clinically practical (one would not surgically straighten one or two remaining toes, for example).

Partial Ray Amputations

The definition of a partial ray amputation is the removal of the toe and part (not all) of the affected metatarsal (Fig. 4). The procedure is performed primarily when

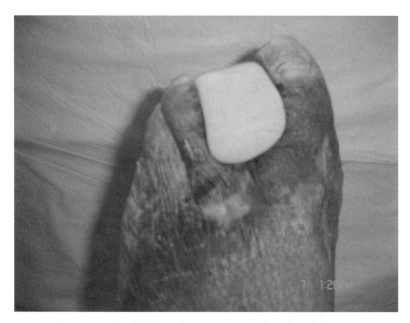

Figure 3 Ortho-digital appliance. Prevents migration of the toes.

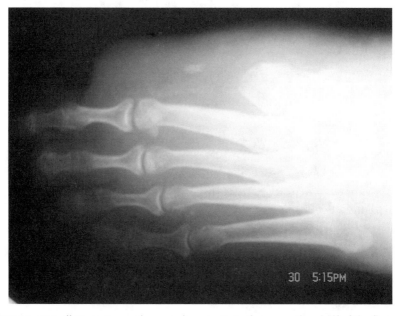

Figure 4 Immediate postoperative x-ray images. Note that more than half of the first metatarsal has been removed.

there is an isolated osteomyelitis affecting the toe(s) and part of the metatarsal(s), abscess with extensive necrosis/gangrene, or trauma.

Single or Isolated Partial Ray Amputations

The weight-bearing portion of a metatarsal is primarily the metatarsal head (MTH). If amputated, the weight borne by the MTH must be dissipated by the remaining architecture of the foot. The consequence is force and stress placed on adjacent bony structures resulting in formation of transfer lesions, fractures, or Charcot destruction similar to that described in the previous digital amputation section (Fig. 5). The degree of weight transfer is dependent on which metatarsals are removed and how much metatarsal remains.

Often, the hardest partial ray amputation to control and the one that ends with the most devastating postoperative results is the 1st ray, especially if more than half of its length is taken. Common sequelae include transfer lesions under the lesser MTHs, fracture of the lesser metatarsals, Charcot osteoarthropathy of the lesser MTPJs or metatarsal-tarsal joints, or subluxation at the metatarsal-tarsal joints. The medial column becomes unstable and the foot becomes more susceptible to pronatory forces.

The 5th ray, because of its low metatarsal declination angle (Fig. 6), bears weight not only at the metatarsal head but along its shaft as well. Thus, partial 5th ray amputations perform well only if the distal-most portion of the metatarsal is removed. If less than two-thirds of the shaft remains, weight is transferred medially to the 4th metatarsal head and proximally to the base of the 5th metatarsal, where hyperkeratosis or ulcerations may occur.

Resection of the central rays (2–4) can lead not only to transfer lesions, but may also cause splaying of the forefoot through interruption of the transverse intermetatarsal ligament (Dannels 1987).

Multiple Partial Ray Amputations

If the 1st ray plus any additional ray, or if more than two lesser rays are amputated, the outcome is poor (Fig. 7). An uncontrollable force is placed on the remainder of the foot and the risk for transfer ulcerations, fractures, or Charcot osteoarthropathy increases significantly.

Clinical Manifestations:

Transfer lesions are one possible clinical manifestation. The removal of the toe and part of a metatarsal creates a significant loss of weight-bearing capacity. The

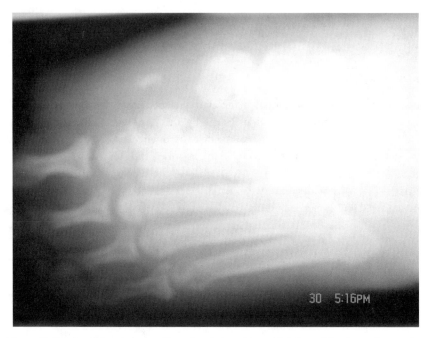

Figure 5 Massive Charcot destruction of metatarsal-tarsal joints and fracture of second metatarsal.

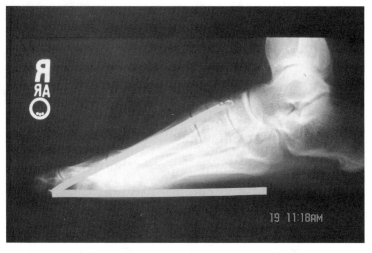

Figure 6 Metatarsal declination angle, seen on an x-ray image of the foot. The term is used to describe the angle created between a metatarsal and the weight-bearing surface. Because the fifth metatarsal creates a small angle, more of its surface touches the ground, bearing more weight.

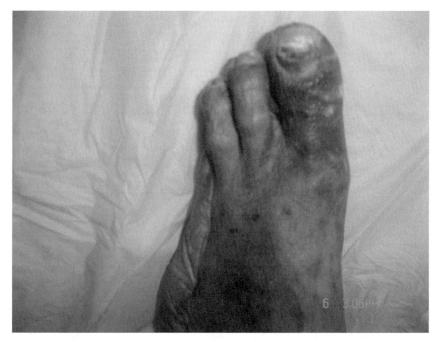

Figure 7 Multiple lesser ray amputations.

weight subsequently is transferred to structures adjacent to the amputated site. As described in the previous sections, this increase in pressure and shear can lead to transfer calluses, ulcerations, fractures, or Charcot osteoarthropathy of neighboring joints. (Charcot osteoarthropathy is very prevalent in this type of amputation. A close clinical watch for changes in size, shape, erythema, or increased warmth of the foot should be performed by both provider and patient.) Bunion deformity, Tailor's bunion deformity, and hammertoe deformity are all possible complications (see Toe Amputation section).

Since more soft tissue support structures are removed with partial ray amputations than with toe amputation, flattening of the arch and widening of the foot can also occur. The extent and speed of flattening of the arch and widening of the foot will depend on the amount of amputation performed.

Treatment

Ortho-digital appliances can be placed in the void of the amputated site (if singular ray amputation) or incorporated into the orthoses (for multiple amputations). These appliances prevent toe drift (see Hallux Amputation Treatment section).

Total contact orthoses are also used. Because this foot is a more complex one to control, it is imperative that the orthoses worn are a total contact variety. They must be fabricated to provide a balance of control for the residual foot and accommodative for any bony prominences or transfer lesion(s). They must be multilayered with the uppermost layer (contacting the patient's skin) made of soft materials, such as, Plastizote-1 and/or poron. The bottom layers can be made of a firmer but not rigid material (such as cork) to provide functional support.

Metatarsal extension modifications can also be made. This modification helps redistribute weight underneath the cut end of the metatarsal. Additional material is incorporated into the orthoses and placed beneath the distal amputation site in order to buttress the load, similar to placing a piece of wood under a short leg of a chair to prevent wobble. The result is a more even distribution of weight that lessens the chance of transfer lesions. Other options include extra-depth or custom-made shoes and padded hosiery (see Hallux Amputation Treatment section).

Surgical correction of digital deformities may also be necessary. Surgical fusion of the remaining toes should be performed only if clinically practical (one would not surgically straighten one or two remaining toes).

Transmetatarsal Amputation

The definition of a transmetatarsal amputation (TMA) is the removal of the entire distal forefoot. Originally described as an amputation performed at the anatomic necks of the five metatarsals, today the surgery is performed anywhere along the metatarsal shafts. The advantages of midfoot amputations include the preservation of normal limb length and the availability of a large, well-padded, weight-bearing surface at the stump end.

Alteration in Gait with Forefoot Amputation

An excellent description of the gait changes seen in proximal foot amputation is offered by Yonclas (Yonclas and O'Donnell 2005):

> Typically the weight progression of the stance leg is from heel to toe with the foot serving as a lever arm for energy absorption and propulsion. In a patient with a partial foot amputation, this progression is altered or absent, and the patient is unable to propel body with the foot during toe-off (Hirsch et al. 1996). As the foot becomes shorter, the ground contact and the functional lever arm of the foot decrease. The residual limb must compensate by

working harder and absorbing more of the ground reaction force, which creates more stress (Catanzarti, Medicino, and Haverstock 1999). In addition, there is an abrupt weight transfer to the opposite limb, which can reduce stride length and velocity resulting in an increase in the energy demands of ambulation. This can lead to increased loads being absorbed on the sound limb with possible increase in degenerative joint changes and subsequent skin breakdown.

To summarize, the gait of a distal foot amputee is as follows:

1. Stride length—shortened on the contralateral limb.
2. More energy expended to walk.
3. Less ability to absorb shock/stress, thus more stress on remaining foot.
4. More stress placed on the contralateral, nonamputated foot.

Thus, the goals of conservative management should focus on the re-establishment of a forefoot lever arm, which will restore a heel-to-toe gait and normal rollover. The result will be decreased stress on both the amputated and nonamputated foot as well as less energy needed for gait.

Clinical Characteristics of TMA

All distal attachments of tendons that dorsiflex the foot are lost with this amputation. The remaining muscle imbalance causes equinovarus deformity: the Achilles and muscles in the posterior compartments of the leg cause the equinus (foot plantarflexed to leg) component of this deformity. The anterior tibialis muscle creates the varus component, forefoot rotated in the frontal plane with the big toe side of the foot higher than the 5th toe side. This places an inordinate amount of pressure on the distal/plantar ridge and/or the plantar-lateral side of the foot. If left uncorrected, the foot continues to drift in the varus direction, making the patient prone to ankle sprains, ankle dislocation, or Charcot. The patient is at high risk for falls.

Clinical manifestations include:

1. Callus underneath the distal cut ends of the metatarsal.
2. Callus or ulcer formation beneath the 5th metatarsal or styloid process.
3. Chronic swelling of the lateral ankle secondary to repeated sprains and/or peroneal tenosynovitis.

Treatment of TMA

The goal of surgical intervention is to prevent equinovarus deformity. Two procedures are effective: tendo-Achilles lengthening (TAL) or an anterior tibialis tendon transfer to the dorsal midfoot. A TAL corrects the equinus component of the deformity. It also prevents the strong pull of the gastroc-soles that overpowers the remaining muscles of the foot from plantarflexing the foot at the ankle.

An anterior tibialis tendon transfer to the dorsal midfoot corrects the varus component of the deformity. By moving the insertion of this tendon laterally, its pull is now more pure dorsiflexion than in a varus direction.

Treatment that is more conservative includes:

1. Custom-molded short shoe with rocker sole. For a foot with compromised vascularity, a patient who is a limited ambulator, or someone with an unsteady gait due to lower extremity weakness, this shoe works best. Patients with poor perfusion usually have atrophic skin, not capable of withstanding a great deal of pressure. The shorter lever arm of this shoe creates less stress on the distal aspect of foot. The rocker sole provides even greater unloading of the distal foot as well as easing roll over, making gait more efficient. The shoe is lighter in weight and affords easier maneuverability and less energy expenditure.

2. Custom-molded regular-length shoe with filler. The filler creates anterior support in the area of the lost metatarsals and a fulcrum around which the foot and ankle pivots during late stance. The result is a more normal/stable gait and less weight transference to the contralateral limb. Care must be taken during fabrication, however, for if the anterior filler is too stiff, an increased pressure on the amputated distal end is applied. Another option is to add an extended steel shank in the sole of the shoe or a carbon foot plate under the orthosis in the shoe. This modification extends from the heel to the ball of the shoe (where the metatarsal heads would have been), replacing the lever arm effect lost by the amputation of the forefoot. This allows the residual foot to advance in a more heel-to-toe fashion, making gait more efficient.

3. A custom-made AFO, such as an Arizona Ankle Brace® or Richie Brace®, is used if significant pronation of the foot is present.

Lisfranc Amputation

Lisfranc amputation is the complete removal of the metatarsals from their tarsal articulations. The indications for this type of amputation are similar to those

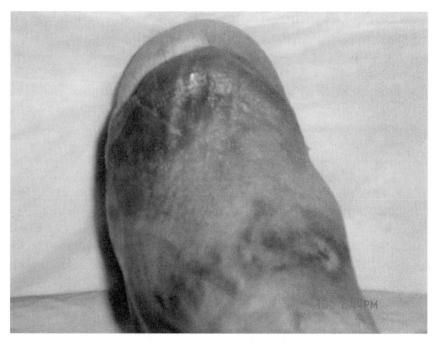

Figure 8 Lisfranc amputation. A TMA would be longer.

described for a TMA except the extent of involvement is greater and more proximal (Fig. 8).

Alterations in gait are even more pronounced in this type of amputation because more musculotendinous attachments are lost. The chance for muscular imbalance, foot instability, and equinovarus deformity postsurgery is significant.

Clinical Characteristics of Lisfranc Amputation

See Clinical Characteristics of TMA section.

Treatment of Lisfranc Amputation

As the foot gets progressively shorter, the changes in gait will become more pronounced. Because the lever arm is so short, the residual foot loses a tremendous amount of ability to absorb and dissipate the force of gait. This increase in stress is directed at the distal aspect of the residual foot. In addition, stride length is further decreased, and the weight transference to the intact limb is even more pronounced. Degenerative joint changes as well as skin breakdown are even more possible.

The goal for conservative management should be to attempt to re-establish as near normal gait as possible. This will result in less stress on the amputated foot as well as the contralateral unaffected limb. Conservative measures include the following options:

1. Custom-molded short shoes with rocker bottom.
2. Custom-molded regular-length shoe with filler, with an extended steel shank or carbon footplate (see Treatment of TMA section).
3. Custom-made AFO if significant pronation of the foot is present.
4. Charcot Restraint Orthotic Walker (CROW) with short or full-length foot section with filler (be aware that the longer the foot section, the greater the shear and ground reactive forces are at the distal plantar surface, which can lead to breakdown).
5. Prosthetic foot. A prosthetic foot supplies little more than cosmetic restoration unless it is modified with materials to provide added support (Yonclas and O'Donnell 2005). It should be used in combination with a custom-molded shoe and should not be used solely as a supportive or functional device.

Surgical options include an Achilles tendon lengthening or an anterior tibialis tendon transfer if varus deformity is noted.

Chopart Amputation

Chopart amputation is the removal of the entire foot save the talus and calcaneus. This amputation creates the most unstable and difficult to control foot postoperatively. The patient is basically balancing on two remaining foot bones with no tendinous attachments except the Achilles. The only supporting structures of these bones are their ligamentous attachments. If no external reinforcing support is provided, in the form of bracing or shoe modification, Charcot or dislocation of the ankle and/or subtalar joint may occur.

Equinovarus formation is very prevalent following this procedure (DeCotiis 2005). There must be a viable heel pad for this procedure to be successful. If there is atrophy or excessive scarring (from previous surgeries) of the heel pad, the results are less than satisfactory. Uncontrollable callus, ulceration, or decubitus-like skin breakdown may occur. This amputation works best for limited ambulators or those who require stability for functional transfers. Because this amputation results in such a short foot, there is an inadequate forefoot lever, which limits push-off and stability. Thus, this is not a procedure for active amputees (Yonclas and O'Donnell 2005).

Clinical Characteristics of Chopart Amputation

Clinical characteristics of a Chopart amputation can be an equinus deformity, a varus deformity, or a Charcot osteoarthropathy. The clinical manifestations of the equinus deformity could include a callus distally, both plantar (from ground reactive forces and shear) and dorsally (from shoe irritation). Varus deformities may manifest as chronic inflammation of the ankle from a soft tissue strain or sprain, or ulceration of the lateral malleolus. The lateral malleolus can become quite prominent if the foot or ankle subluxes and goes into severe inversion. The clinical manifestations of a Charcot osteoarthropathy include a red, hot, swollen ankle with abnormal range of motion (decreased or significantly increased) and crepitus.

Treatment of Chopart Amputation

Surgical treatment of a Chopart amputation includes either a TAL or a more proximal amputation (below- or above-knee amputation). A more conservative treatment would be to provide the patient with a Charcot Restraint Orthotic Walker (CROW). This device provides a short or full-length shoe with filler to help the patient ambulate.

Summary

Subtotal foot amputations are sometimes an inevitable result of diabetic complications and should not be looked upon as treatment failures but rather as limb salvage procedures that maintain the greatest possible functional capability and ambulatory power for the patient. The long-term success following amputation is inevitably the responsibility of the team of clinicians and patient educators providing care as well as a committed participatory patient. Anticipating clinical manifestations for each level of amputation will arm the provider and patient with early warning signs that, if identified and treated aggressively and expeditiously, will help prevent ulceration, infection, and further amputation.

References

Catanzarti AR, Medicino RW, Haverstock B. Considerations for protection of the residual following transmetatarsal amputation. *Wounds* 11:13–20, 1999.

Dannels, EG. Prevention of complications of partial foot amputations. *Clin Pod Med Surg* 4:503–516, 1987.

DeCotiis, MA. Lisfranc and Chopart amputations. *Clin Pod Med Surg* 20:385–393, 2005.

Hirsch G, McBride ME, Murray DD, Sanderson DJ, Dukes I, Menard MR. Chopart prosthesis and semirigid foot orthosis in traumatic forefoot amputation: Comparative gait analysis. *Am J Phys Med Rehabil* 75:283–291, 1996.

Levin M. Preventing amputation in the patient with diabetes. *Diabetes Care* 18:1383–1391, 1995.

Moore, JW. Prostheses, orthoses, and shoes for partial foot amputees. *Clin Pod Med Surg* 14:775–783, 1997.

Poppen NK, Mann RA, O'Konski M, Buncke HJ. Amputation of the great toe. *Foot Ankle* 1:333–337, 1981.

Pulla, RJ, Kaminsky, KM. Toe amputations and ray resections. *Clin Pod Med Surg* 14:691–729, 1997.

Quebedeaux T, Lavery L, Lavery D. The development of foot deformities and ulcers after great toe amputation in diabetes. *Diabetes Care* 19:165–167, 1996.

Stuck, RM, Sage, R, Pinzur, M, Osterman, H. Amputations in the diabetic foot. *Clin Pod Med Surg* 12:141–155, 1995.

Veves A, Masson E, Fernando D, Boulton AJM. Use of experimental padded hosiery to reduce abnormal foot pressures in diabetic neuropathy. *Diabetes Care* 12:653–655, 1989.

Yonclas PP, O'Donnell CJ. Prosthetic management of the partial foot amputee. *Clin Pod Med Surg* 22:485–502, 2005.

Suggested Readings

Bowker JH, Pfeifer MA. *Levin and O'Neal's The Diabetic Foot*, 6th ed. St. Louis, Mosby 2001.

Kominsky SJ: *Medical and Surgical Management of the Diabetic Foot*. St. Louis, Mosby 1994.

4

Major Leg Amputation

Bertram E. Feingold, MD

Introduction

Wars have always been a training ground for the surgeon, and the same is true for the treatment of severe war wounds that devitalize the extremity, requiring amputation. It wasn't until World War II that a large number of amputations done successfully necessitated the high demand for achieving a good relationship between the residual limb and a well-performing prosthesis. During the 1940s, a great deal of early research began into the development of better performing lower extremity prostheses. The study of biomechanics along with the improving surgical techniques and postoperative rehabilitation techniques allowed marked improvement in amputation results and thus began an explosive development in higher performing prosthetics over the second half of the 20th century.

Today, amputations should be performed by surgeons who have an interest in and a complete understanding of the disease process and an understanding of the current principles of amputation surgery. This, combined with knowledge of the patient's overall health status and personal goals, is necessary in order to plan a postoperative rehabilitation program and eventual fabrication of the artificial limb by a prosthetist. Amputations are reconstructive procedures and should be considered as a part of the plan to return a patient to a more comfortable and productive life.

In the history of medicine, the initial etiology for lower extremity amputations was trauma, especially wars. Today, particularly in the Western world, the etiology has changed to peripheral vascular disease and diabetes. In the early 1900s, only 2% or 3% of amputations were attributable to peripheral vascular disease, but by the mid-20th century peripheral vascular disease accounted for over 50% of all amputations. There is a rising number of amputations being performed each year primarily because of the aging population. In the Western world today, over 90% of amputations are related to peripheral vascular disease. However, in the younger populations, trauma and malignancy are the leading causes for amputation surgery (Heck and Carnesale 2003). In the 21st century, about 50%–70% of the patients with peripheral vascular disease that necessitates amputation through the lower extremity have diabetes mellitus.

Amputation today, although recognized as one of the most ancient of all operations, also remains one of the most frequent procedures done, particularly in the diabetic population. There are estimated to be more than 400,000 amputees in the United States, of which the majority are in the lower extremity (McCollough 1986). Because the majority of lower extremity amputations are related to peripheral vascular disease, complications of the surgery are usually related to ischemic problems.

Why Amputate

Amputations are done for a pathological state that often results in loss of function and may even be life-threatening. In a situation where there is uncontrollable infection, amputation may be necessary as a life-preserving measure. Likewise, in the case of tumor, amputation may be life-saving, but with newer techniques limb-sparing operations are often performed. The basic goal of an amputation surgeon is to eliminate the pathological process and restore the function that is being prevented by the pathology at hand. Many times the need for surgery may be severe infection that is not controllable or is irreversible. Other times, the need might be severe pain from ischemia, infection, or deformity. Certain congenital anomalies of the lower extremity may also be an etiology for amputation. Therefore, amputation surgery should be considered reconstructive surgery that eliminates the disease process and, with prosthetic replacement, restores function to the highest possible level. This may be merely mobilizing the patient from bed to chair or restoration of ambulation.

Population at Risk

In the diabetic patient, the most frequent site for an infection begins somewhere in the foot. Usually the soft tissues undergo some type of breakdown (Coleman and Brand 1997). Frequently, these are on the plantar aspect of the foot or over some bony prominence such as the inner border of the great toe or on the tops of the toes from rubbing against the inside of a shoe. In a diabetic patient, there is often a combination of neuropathy and the loss of sensation. Thus, the insensate foot, unable to detect when there is violation of the skin, is vulnerable to rapidly developing infection. Often with neuropathy, there may be peripheral vascular impairment. Vascular disease may be present in a diabetic patient with or without symptoms (Levin, Sicard, and Rubin 1997). Failure to treat an ingrown toenail or skin ulceration early will result in subsequent infection that can quickly spread throughout the foot. With impaired circulation, it becomes difficult to deliver appropriate antibiotic medication. Therefore, subsequent infection and/or gangrene may develop, necessitating amputation. The diabetic foot with neuropathy is a foot at risk for skin breakdown and bacterial infection. The normal nondiabetic patient without neuropathy would not be able to tolerate weight bearing due to severe pain from any skin violation or infection. However, the neuropathic foot is essentially insensate and thus the patient fails to note the early onset of a problem until it becomes obvious when the patient develops severe swelling, fever, chills, redness, or drainage.

Early action, such as frequent examination of the feet, is extremely important to prevent these problems from occurring. Once an early breakdown in the skin occurs or an ingrown toenail starts to develop, appropriate action must be taken and the problem brought to the attention of the treating physician. The patient with a diabetic foot, as the years go by, has progressive loss of sensation and an ever-increasing risk for unrecognized trauma occurring. Early consultation with an orthotist regarding use of protective and accommodative footwear will reduce much of the destructive, unrecognized stress to the feet. Therefore, it is imperative that both feet are examined daily for any signs of skin breakdown or increased swelling, discoloration, or redness. If observed this must be reported immediately to the patient's treating physician.

Unfortunately, peripheral vascular disease is very common in the diabetic patient after age 50 and often results in complications that result in an amputation. Peripheral vascular disease in a diabetic patient is not necessarily limited to the involved extremity but may also involve other areas such as the cerebrovascular supply, coronary artery supply, and the renal blood supply. In diabetes mellitus, peripheral vascular disease consists of a microvascular component that results in nephropathy and retinopathy, and a macrovascular component that will often result in peripheral arterial disease, stroke, and heart attacks (myocardial infarction). Diabetic and nondiabetic patients have the same pathological process involving the vessel walls. However, in a diabetic patient onset of the pathological process occurs at a younger age and accelerates more rapidly. In diabetes, men and women have the same rate of occurrence of this process while in the nondiabetic population peripheral vascular disease is more common in men than women.

In the nondiabetic population, the vessels involved are usually the abdominal aorta, and the iliac and femoral vessels above the knee, while in the diabetic population the usual involvement is below the knee, where the smaller vessels such as the tibialis and peroneal arteries and their distal branches are located. In addition, the diabetic patient most likely has bilateral lower extremity involvement with multiple levels of involvement of the proximal and distal vessels. In a nondiabetic patient, involvement usually is unilateral and includes a single segment as opposed to the multisegment levels in the diabetic patient. Routine X-rays of the lower extremities and feet in diabetic patients will frequently demonstrate vascular calcifications as far distal as the toes. This is visual confirmation of the deposition of lipids, cholesterol, and calcification in the walls of the blood vessels. The small vessel calcifications confirm the microvascular component of diabetes mellitus. In spite of these calcifications, there may still be palpable pulses in the feet of some diabetic patients.

Preoperative Medical Evaluation

With the diabetic foot that is at risk for infection with nonhealing areas of skin breakdown, it is important to get a preoperative medical workup to determine the degree of vascular insufficiency in that extremity. This includes an extensive medical workup because the pathophysiology of diabetes involves multiple systems including the heart, brain, kidneys, and peripheral nerves and vessels. At times, vascular involvement is so extensive that there is vascular compromise in the upper extremities as well, including the distal tips of fingers that will occasionally present with nonhealing ulcerations.

Tests such as arterial Doppler studies can be done to determine the presence or absence of pulses and the waveforms of the pulse, and are extremely important in the arterial evaluation of the diabetic patient. There can be pedal pulses in the presence of extensive disease in the tibial and peroneal vessels. However, segmental systolic blood pressures can be misleading and falsely elevated due to the atherosclerotic vessels and the false elevation of the readings with noncompliant vascular walls. There are a number of skin perfusion tests such as thermography, laser Doppler flowmetry, or injection of substances like fluorescein and

Xenon 133. However, a more practical and reliable test seems to be the transcutaneous oxygen measurements (TCOM study) in multiple sites along an extremity. It is important to get the measurement performed in room air and again after breathing 100% oxygen. If there is an improvement of the oxygen saturation by 10 mm while breathing 100% oxygen, then this is a good indicator for potential wound healing. The test can be misleading (and falsely interpreted) because of oxygen diffusion problems in the presence of edema and cellulitis.

A comprehensive evaluation of the lower extremity vascular system is best determined with a vascular surgery consultation. Revascularization of the involved extremity will often improve the rate of ulcer healing or result in an amputation to perhaps a more distal level. Arteriograms are often helpful in determining the possibility for angioplasty of the vessels (dilation and distention of the narrowed areas plus options for possible insertion of a stent to hold the vessel open). The arteriogram also provides information to the vascular surgeon if there is a possibility for bypass surgery to improve distal perfusion, particularly in problems where there are nonhealing ulcers and infection in the foot and ankle region.

The preoperative workup should also include an extensive assessment of the patient's general medical condition. Simple tests for nutritional status and immunological competence should be performed. All medical illnesses including any underlying infection should be brought under control. Correcting these conditions will reduce the chance of perioperative complications. Malnourishment increases the rate of postoperative complications, particularly wound healing. Simple observation such as the color of the skin, hair growth or absence thereof, and skin temperatures of the extremity provide invaluable information as to the prognosis for wound healing.

During amputation surgery, skin edge bleeding is a good prognosticator for healing. Should bleeding be poor or minimal at best, a higher-level amputation may be indicated.

Planning the Amputation Level

Determination of the amputation level is multifactorial. After identification and correction of the previously mentioned medical problems and vascular status of the extremity, then the level of amputation is considered (Fig. 1). This includes, of course, the health status of the patient and his ambulatory potential. If there is no ambulatory potential, then the primary goal is to achieve the highest probability for wound healing with decreased perioperative morbidity. However, if there is ambulatory potential, then it is the surgeon's goal to achieve the most distant level for amputation with the most reasonable chance for healing. This is due to the energy cost of walking for patients with amputations. Studies have revealed

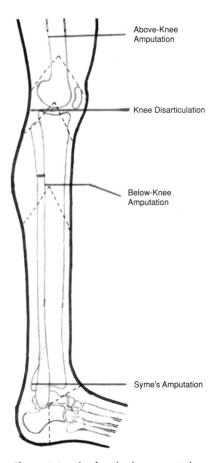

Figure 1 Levels of major leg amputation.

that the higher the level of amputation, the greater energy expended while the lower the level of amputation, the more likely the return to ambulatory activities. Thus, the surgeon always attempts to perform the lowest possible level of amputation consistent with a reasonable chance for successful healing and the lowest risk of complications.

Recognizing that salvaging the foot is the primary goal, then any early invasion of infection or development of ulcerations and skin breakdown on the foot becomes of grave concern to all who treat the diabetic patient. If there is infection in the foot, then the depth and extent of that infection must be determined. Routine X-rays and advanced imaging studies such as technetium-99m bone scan, indium labeled leukocyte scan, computed tomography scan, and magnetic resonance imaging scan are often part of the workup to make this determination.

Any involvement of the deep soft tissues and bones in the foot must be diagnosed to plan the preoperative medical care and subsequent surgical management. If blood flow is adequate, then simple local wound care is sometimes aggressively performed by surgeons to eliminate the chronic infected and necrotic tissue, which allows drainage and healing of the wound. Consultation with physicians who have expertise in treatment of infections to select and direct the antibiotic therapy program is also advised. Again, it is the intent of the surgeon treating the foot to save as much of that anatomical structure as possible. Even different levels of partial foot amputations from the toes to the midfoot result in successful salvage procedures and, if accomplished, near normal ambulation can be restored with today's modern materials and techniques of shoe fabrication and orthotics. On the other hand, once a decision that foot salvage is not possible and amputation proximal to the heel is necessary, then planning for the next higher level of amputation is undertaken. Again, the surgeon needs to maximize the opportunity to achieve the lowest level of amputation with the highest degree of successful wound healing and achieving the goal of eliminating the pathological process and resuming ambulation.

Determination of the level of amputation above the foot (foot being defined as distal to the talus and calcaneus) depends on the condition of the vascular supply along with good nutrition and the absence of any issues of skin viability. The preoperative information of oxygen perfusion from the TCOM study, distal arterial vascular flow from the arteriogram, the absence of any issues about skin viability and no adjacent infections would hopefully indicate the level to be through the ankle joint. This level is known as a Syme's amputation and is considered the most effective and easiest level of amputation for ambulation. Syme's amputations, however, seem to be technically difficult for many surgeons to accomplish. Successful healing can be difficult to achieve as noted earlier. As the years pass, progression of the peripheral vascular disease often occurs in the involved lower extremity resulting in skin breakdown in the stump and failure to heal. This may necessitate conversion of the Syme's amputation to the next higher level or transtibial amputation.

The most common and frequently planned leg amputation above the foot is the transtibial level, also known as the below-knee amputation (BKA). This also is a very gait-efficient level and most patients ambulating preoperatively can resume ambulation with a proper-fitting prosthesis. Preservation of the knee joint with a healthy proximal transtibial amputation (about 4–6 inches long) is the surgeon's goal.

Other levels of successful lower extremity amputation include knee disarticulation and transfemoral above-knee amputation (AKA). Knee disarticulation describes exactly that, amputation through the knee joint and removal of the tibia, leaving the patella intact and preserving the entire length of the femur to give a long lever arm for sitting balance and maximizing the mechanical efficiency of the quadriceps and hamstring muscles. The end bearing of the knee disarticulation surgery is excellent. The AKA levels likewise are excellent for prosthetic usage, but again, there is a higher degree of energy utilization the more proximal the amputation. Thus for the elderly diabetic patient an AKA requires much greater effort to resume ambulation.

General Surgical Principles

General technical aspects of an amputation operation include observing the principles of gentle soft tissue handling to enhance good wound healing. Avoidance of excessively long soft tissue flaps and flap traumatization reduces the risk of potential wound healing problems. Skin flaps that are created should be full thickness and not undermined. They should be closed without tension on the suture line. Painful scar formation in the soft tissue flaps should be avoided, particularly adherence of the skin to bone, because this can make comfortable fitting of the prosthesis difficult. Achieving good hemostasis at the time of surgery is of utmost importance. Often a tourniquet is used during surgery to reduce bleeding. The tourniquet should be released prior to wound closure to inspect the wound and secure hemostasis before closure. Secure ligation of isolated larger vessels is important as well as meticulous control of the smaller vessels with ligation and cautery. The wound should be drained for 48–72 hours following surgery. The nerves exposed at the operative site should be isolated. All nerves that are cut form a healing scar called a neuroma. The nerves should be gently pulled distally, cut with a knife, and then allowed to retract proximal to the ends of the bone resection. The bone ends should be trimmed square, beveled, and rasped to achieve smooth contours and then padded with soft tissue coverage. Smooth contours should be achieved by rasping the ends. Excessive subperiosteal stripping should be avoided to prevent devitalization of the bone and later possible development of bony overgrowth (bone spurs).

Some extremities will present with skin and soft tissue destruction from trauma and/or infection close to the level of the planned amputation. This may necessitate delayed wound closure techniques. In patients with massive extremity infection, performing an open (guillotine) procedure may be a life-saving operation. Definitive wound debridement and repair would be performed a few days later. In less severely infected limbs, such as those with cellulitis and possibly skin ulceration close to the planned skin incisions, performing the surgery but not closing the wound definitively is advised. This would be a temporary or partial closure of the soft tissues with re-evaluation of the operative area for residual infection and ischemia in two to three days. Occasionally further soft tissue removal is required due to the previously mentioned reasons and even a higher level of bone amputation required to permit adequate soft tissue closure without tension.

Levels of Lower Leg Amputation Surgery

Syme's amputation (disarticulation through the ankle) is a lower leg amputation that best preserves lower extremity function and minimizes disability (Pinzur et al. 2003) but is not very popular among amputation surgeons (Fig. 2). A high level of wound complications is reported with this procedure and thus many surgeons avoid the Syme's amputation. This operation involves a simple ankle disarticulation (removal of the entire foot through the talotibial joint) and

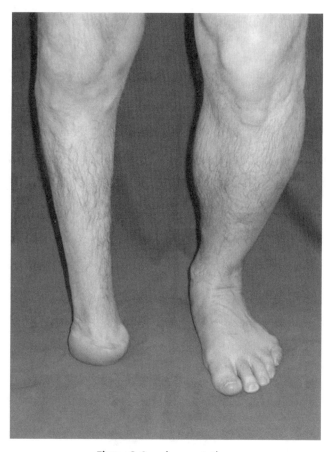

Figure 2 Syme's amputation.

preserving the heel pad. The distal tibia articular surface and both medial and lateral malleoli are osteotomized (cut) at 90 degrees to the tibial axis and just proximal to the concavity of the distal tibia articular surface. Then the heel pad is rotated and sutured into place over the distal tibia. The most common causes for unsatisfactory Syme's amputations are posterior heel pad migration, infection, and skin slough from trimming the skin edges too vigorously. Success depends on meticulous surgical technique and delayed weight bearing until the limb heals securely. Heel pad migration makes fitting of a prosthesis very difficult if not impossible.

The Syme's prosthesis tends to be bulky where it fits over the flare of the distal tibia. For women this may present particular concern regarding appearance. However, there are described techniques to reduce the flare surgically to slightly larger than the diaphyseal region of the distal tibia. This allows an improved appearance of the prosthesis (smaller appearance at the ankle). Functionally the Syme's level amputation is extremely good. Most patients can return to their pre-amputation level of activity. The energy cost for walking with this prosthesis is the most efficient of all lower extremity major amputations. Another small but important bonus from this level is that it usually permits weight bearing and limited ambulation without a prosthesis. This can be important for nighttime trips to the bathroom because it avoids the need to put on a prosthesis before stepping out of bed. All other higher levels of amputations require application of a prosthesis or use of an ambulatory aid (walkers, crutches, or wheelchair) in order to get up from bed. At night, amputees, especially older people, may forget to apply their prosthesis and simply stepping out of bed can result in a fall and the risk of serious injury. The Syme's amputee would have less risk for a fall and injury.

The most frequent and very successful level of lower extremity amputation, particularly for patients with peripheral vascular disease, has been transtibial amputations (upper one-third of the tibia, called BKA; Fig. 3). In the nonischemic limb, the ideal level is below the knee at the musculotendinous junction of the gastrocnemius muscle. The tibia cut is about 15 cm distal to the articular surface of the tibia (the fibula 1–2 cm shorter) with the soft tissue flaps much more distal. In nonischemic extremities the skin and muscle flaps are closed, usually with tension myodesis and myoplasty techniques. This means suturing muscles to bone (myodesis) with tension such as to the tibia or femur and/or suturing muscles to muscles (myoplasty with tension such as quadriceps repaired to the hamstrings). More efficient muscle function can then be achieved during the rehabilitation program. However, tension cannot be tolerated in the ischemic limb and often the bone amputation levels are higher at about 10–12 cm and without tension myodesis or myoplasty. The blood supply is usually better in the posterior flaps and thus in the ischemic limb, there is often a longer posterior flap sutured to the

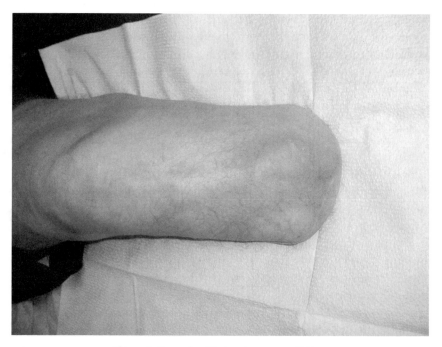

Figure 3 Example of below-knee amputation.

anterior flap while in the nonischemic limb the flaps are often equal anteriorly and posteriorly or medially and laterally. Flap design is often determined by the particular wound problems at the time of surgery and where the better blood supply is located. Surgery is usually done in the nonischemic limb with a tourniquet. In the severely ischemic limb with prior vascular surgery, the use of a tourniquet is often contraindicated. Nevertheless, hemostasis is important in either situation and this must be secured prior to wound closure.

Suction surgical drains are placed in the wound and exit proximal to the amputation level. The drains should remove much of the postoperative blood loss from deep inside the closed incision and prevent increased internal wound pressure from developing. If that were to occur, then ischemia to the deep tissues and even skin could cause failure of the flaps to heal. Drains are usually removed at 48–72 hours after surgery. The extremity is dressed with a soft compressive type of dressing. Some physicians prefer a thin cast application (postoperative rigid dressing) over this from the cut end to the proximal thigh. The cast is often molded over the supracondylar region and a suspension strap is applied to prevent the cast from slipping. This is an excellent technique to prevent a flexion contracture from developing at the knee. The knee is flexed about 5–10 degrees to reduce the tension on the posterior hamstring muscles. The rigid dressing also affords mild compression to the wound to reduce edema and tension on the suture line. Immobilizing the residual limb helps to reduce pain from motion at the knee and facilitates transfers from bed to chair immediately after surgery. With a strap around the waist to the cast, there is good suspension of the rigid dressing for standing activities. The cast can be changed between five to seven days, particularly if it becomes loose. Some physicians prefer to completely remove the cast by seven days and place the limb in a removable splint with a stump sock or compression dressing. Wound healing must be adequate, particularly on the ischemic extremity, and in diabetic patients before weight bearing is allowed. This is to be determined by the surgeon and may be as much as six to eight weeks after surgery when the edema has resolved and the wound edges have completely healed. Sutures sometimes are allowed to remain in the wound four to six weeks depending on any underlying healing problems. Once the prosthesis is produced and fitted by the prosthetist and a rehabilitation program completed, the large majority of patients with transtibial amputations will successfully learn to use their prosthesis and ambulate again. See Chapter 7 for further discussion on post-op rigid dressings.

Disarticulation of the knee is an excellent level of amputation if it is not possible to salvage a below-knee level due to insufficient soft tissue coverage (Fig. 4). However, in older patients, there is sometimes concern for ischemia in the long flaps and this should be taken into consideration and avoided if there is a possibility of necrosis. The advantage of this level of amputation is the excellent end-bearing surface of the distal femur and patella covered with skin. This provides a long lever arm that allows the hamstrings and quadriceps muscles to work more efficiently. Also, the prosthesis fitting is often more stable due to its length of contact. Newer techniques with prosthetic knee mechanisms and suspension techniques are now making this a more feasible level of amputation, although it is not as popular as the AKA in most surgeons' repertoire. For the nonambulatory patient, this also is an ideal level because it provides a longer lever arm for sitting balance and support and avoids complications of knee flexion contracture and distal stump ulcers in nonfunctional below-knee amputees.

The next level of amputation is the transfemoral or AKA (Fig. 5). Once again, it is desirable to attempt to provide as long a limb as possible to enhance prosthetic fitting and control. Amputation should usually be done approximately 10 cm or so above the distal femur to accommodate the knee unit of an above-knee prosthesis. This is for cosmetic purposes and not necessarily for function. In a nonischemic lower extremity, myodesis techniques are important for enhancing muscle stabilization and to ensure a good strong functional limb. However, in the ischemic limb myodesis is to be avoided due to increased risk of injuring the already compromised vascular supply. Still it is important to loosely attach the

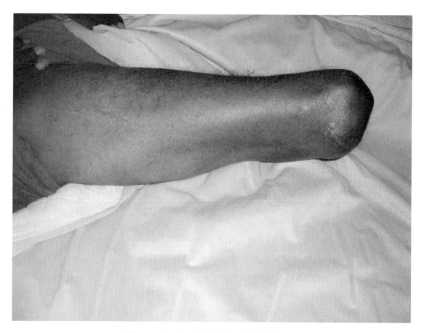

Figure 4 Disarticulation of the knee.

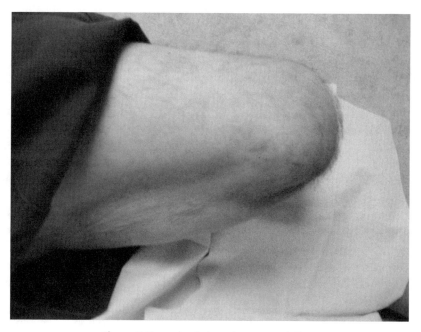

Figure 5 Example of above-knee amputation.

muscles to the femur and attempt to prevent drift of the muscles from the femoral shaft. Stabilizing the muscles helps retain function of the hip flexors, extensors, and adductors. Following wound closure with suction drains for 48–72 hours, a soft compression dressing is applied and once again the wound is inspected regularly and mild compression dressings are exchanged to control edema. About five to seven days after amputation, if possible, a compression sock ("stump" shrinker) is applied. Following wound healing, between six and eight weeks, a prosthesis is fitted and ambulation initiated.

Complications of Amputation Surgery

Complications can occur after lower extremity amputation. One of the earliest problems to develop can be the formation of a hematoma in the wound. This can cause considerable tension under the soft tissues and compromise blood flow with resultant necrosis of the flaps (skin, subcutaneous, and muscle layers). This could then lead to delayed wound healing and wound separation. To avoid this risk, meticulous intraoperative wound management is necessary to control hemostasis, particularly after release of a tourniquet if used and before final wound closure. Drains can reduce this complication. Sometimes a hematoma can develop from bleeding secondary to anticoagulation needed postoperatively, which can result in large subcutaneous or deep muscle bleeding. Aspiration of the hematoma is a possibility or occasionally it is necessary to return to the operating room for evacuation of the hematoma and inspection for any continual bleeding sites.

Wound dehiscence or separation is particularly common in patients with vascular disease. This can occur from premature removal of sutures or where there is some necrosis of the skin edges. Avoidance of this can sometimes be achieved with careful subcutaneous wound closure to reduce tension on the skin line. Removal of skin sutures should be delayed three to four weeks or as long as necessary in patients where there is concern for residual wound ischemia. Likewise, weight bearing in a prosthesis prior to full wound healing should be avoided. Occasionally, acute wound dehiscence, if discovered early, can be closed immediately. Usually this complication would necessitate use of techniques such as delayed wound healing or vacuum-assisted wound closure. Any attempt at delayed wound closure surgically needs to be done so that suturing can be achieved without tension. Today techniques like vacuum-assisted wound closure are utilized to approximate the wound edges. During this period of delayed wound healing, antibiotics are frequently utilized to reduce the risk of bone infection (osteomyelitis).

Unfortunately, gangrene can occur in the postamputation limb. This is associated with full-thickness necrosis of the skin flaps. Occasionally the underlying subcutaneous tissues and muscle layers become necrotic due to progressive ischemia from more proximal vessel occlusion. It is important to observe bleeding from the skin and underlying muscles at the time of surgery. If bleeding is inadequate, particularly after the tourniquet is released, then a higher level of amputation needs to be considered at that time. Skin necrosis along the margins of the flaps can occasionally occur and if it is minimal (1–2 mm), then patience and local wound care will often result in successful healing. If necrosis is extensive beyond 1.2 cm or so, and involving deeper tissues, then surgical debridement is needed to remove the dead tissues along with the use of vacuum-assisted techniques to help close the wound. Occasionally soft tissue loss is so extensive that a higher amputation level is required.

Pressure necrosis can likewise occur from rigid dressings with inadequate padding over bony prominences such as the anterior distal end of the tibia, which is covered with only a very thin layer of skin. If discovered early and the lesion is small, this can often heal with wound care techniques described earlier. If healing fails and/or the wound slowly enlarges, then a higher level of amputation may be required.

Postoperative wound infection is another complication, particularly in patients with preoperative chronic distal infection and/or an acute infection with cellulitis close to the level of amputation. Therefore, consideration for delayed wound closure is appropriate particularly if there is concern for contamination of lymphatics and possible ischemic tissues that may remain in the operative area. Perioperative antibiotics should be used. Postoperative infection can be superficial or deep and often requires consultation with an infectious disease specialist. If the infection is deep and involves bone, then often re-operation is required for extensive soft tissue and bone debridement. Re-amputation is sometimes necessary to resolve this complication.

Wound edema can be serious by causing delay in wound healing and can result in progressive skin ischemia and necrosis. This should be controlled with elevation of the extremity postoperatively and compressive wrappings on the wound. The use of compression socks is often effective in reducing limb swelling. Circular bandages can be dangerous, particularly if they become constrictive proximally and subsequently enhance the edema with a tourniquet-like effect. This reduces arterial blood flow into and venous flow out of the residuum distally. Occasionally the edema can be associated with simultaneous edema in the other extremity. This may be fluid retention secondary to other underlying medical problems like cardiac, renal, or hepatic failure and require appropriate medical treatment to resolve the edema problem.

Additional complications include pain following surgery, which is not unusual and is often controlled with appropriate analgesic medication. However, extreme pain out of proportion to the expected amount should alert the surgeon to evaluate the wound and extremity for possible ischemia/compartment syndrome and treat accordingly. Contractures in the amputated extremity present problems for later ambulation with a prosthesis. In BKAs, flexion contractures at the knee can make prosthetic fitting and utilization more difficult. Likewise at the hip joint flexion, adduction and/or abduction contractures will create problems for above-knee prosthetic fitting and ambulation. Aggressive and early postoperative physical therapy will usually prevent the contractures from occurring. If the contractures are chronic (present prior to amputation) and resistant to physical therapy efforts, then surgical release of the contracture(s) may be indicated in order to effectively fit and utilize a prosthesis. This would involve doing tendon releases when indicated, and if there is still restricted motion, then performing a capsulotomy (open release of the joint capsule) of the involved joint might be necessary. See Chapter 8 for discussion on preventing contractures.

For BKAs, the use of rigid dressings will help prevent knee flexion contractures, or if present preoperatively, reduce the risk of progressive contracture formation. Immobilization of the knee in extension helps prevent this problem, particularly if used for up to two weeks. Pain and muscle spasms after surgery often result in contracture of the knee. Casting the knee in 5–10 degrees of flexion reduces tension on the posterior hamstrings and gastrocnemius muscles, particularly in older people with underlying osteoarthritis. Significant knee flexion contractures can make prosthesis utilization more difficult and less biomechanically efficient.

Late complications can occur in the diabetic patient. The loss of one limb to ischemia and diabetes results in approximately a 20%–50% chance of the remaining leg requiring amputation within five years. Local complications of the residual limb occasionally develop. Skin problems occasionally occur when the prosthesis no longer fits properly (too tight or too loose). This will cause skin irritation, abrasions, blistering, and fissuring of the skin. During the first year, the residual limb will atrophy and shrink at varying rates. With a diabetic patient, impaired sensation may be present from the underlying peripheral neuropathy and thus unrecognized skin irritations can develop. Weight loss and atrophy will often change the contact surfaces between the limb and socket with development of end bearing on the stump and then progressive skin breakdown. This is common on the distal and anterior crest of the tibia and sometimes over the fibular head. Weight gain can cause limb volume to increase and improper fitting. Occasionally malalignment of the prosthesis can result in excess pressure on the residuum. On the other hand, inadequate beveling of the anterior crest of the tibia can cause unsolvable problems of skin necrosis necessitating surgical revision.

Additional, less frequent complications include painful scars that can occur with amputations requiring delayed wound healing techniques. This may occur with acute infections where guillotine-type amputations are performed that require vacuum suction techniques to close the wound. Edema problems or skin irritation from eczema or folliculitis can present from time to time. Excessive soft tissue at the end of the limb occasionally requires surgical excision. Bony prominences at the end of the amputation site with inadequate soft tissue coverage often can present delayed problems with ulcerations. Occasionally a bone spur confirmed by X-ray and local tenderness will develop. Initial treatment is conservative: a socket adjustment, local injection with steroid, and if these fail, then surgical excision.

Residual pain is one of the more common complications from amputation surgery. Sometimes this is due to pain in the residuum itself such as from a neuroma. Neuroma formation occurs in every transected nerve, but if the nerve is left in an unprotected area where there is major contact, then a burning type of paresthesias can occur and this often requires adjustment of the prosthesis. Additional treatments for a symptomatic neuroma might be a steroid and lidocaine injection into the neuroma region, which sometimes relieves the pain temporarily or long term. The best method of treatment for neuromas is usually surgical excision, nerve ligation, and burying the nerve end deep into soft tissues or even bone. Sometimes fabrication of a new prosthetic socket may be needed to relieve pressure at the neuroma area and resolve the pain.

Some patients will develop a bursa over bony prominences like the end of the amputated bone. This is a normal physiological process but sometimes the bursa can become inflamed from excessive pressure. Treatment can be physical therapy, local injection, oral anti-inflammatory medications, prosthetic adjustment, and occasionally, surgical excision of the bursa.

Nerve compression from the prosthetic socket: the sciatic nerve in AKAs, and the peroneal nerve in the BKA can cause diffuse stump pain and parenthesis. Socket adjustment is the usual treatment of choice. Still another cause of pain is proximal nerve root compression resulting from a lumbar disc herniation. Treatment may require epidural nerve blocks or surgery for the removal of the source of the nerve root compression.

Lower extremity ischemia can reoccur over time as the peripheral vascular disease slowly progresses. Skin changes in the amputated limb such as color, temperature (coldness), and hypersensitivity may suggest developing arterial occlusion. Also, vascular claudication symptoms may develop when ambulating in the prosthesis (i.e., buttock, thigh, or leg cramping relieved with rest). These symptoms require further vascular evaluation.

Phantom limb pain is another complication of amputation surgery that is usually transient. It can be very incapacitating for a small minority of patients. There is a distinction between phantom pain and phantom limb. Phantom limb (present in 85% to 90% of patients) is a sensation that the limb is still present and often is described as a sensation of tingling. It is usually associated with a gradual decline in the sensation, and the tingling feeling disappears in most cases. Phantom pain occurs in about 35% of amputees but is debilitating much less frequently, at about 5%–10%. This phenomenon is more common in patients with chronic pain in the limb before amputation. Characteristics of phantom pain are cramping or squeezing pain, burning pain, and sharp or shooting pain. Etiology of phantom pain may be from the peripheral or central nervous system. Another theory is that psychogenic factors may contribute to this phenomenon. Treatment of phantom pain is wide and varied. Many different medications, physical therapy such as ultrasound and electrical stimulation, and psychotherapy may be utilized. There are even surgical procedures to remove the source of objective pain that might perpetuate phantom pain such as bony spurs, scars, or neuroma. Higher level of amputation is often not successful. Neurosurgical procedures have been tried such as proximal neurotomy, posterior rhizotomy, anterolateral cordotomy, sympathectomy, postcentral gyrectomy, frontal lobotomy, and thalamotomy. With all the varieties of treatment, it is obvious that no one treatment form is consistently getting good results. See Chapter 10 for more discussion on phantom phenomena.

Causalgia or reflex sympathetic dystrophy (RSD) occasionally occurs in the amputated limb, particularly in the ankle or below-knee levels. Treatment is with sympathetic nerve blocks and special medications. This symptom complex occurs more frequently in patients with labile emotional personalities. If the sympathetic nerve blocks are successful but temporary then surgical sympathectomy can be performed with lasting results.

Summary

Patients needing an amputation today most often have severe peripheral vascular disease with associated diabetes mellitus. Unfortunate and often unrecognized trauma (injury) occurs to the lower extremity (especially the foot), resulting in failure to heal and subsequent development of increasingly painful infection and even gangrene. Once this develops, the patient's functional capacity rapidly declines and life and limb suddenly can be in jeopardy requiring emergency amputations. According to Robert Tooms 1987, EM Burgess, a well-known orthopedic amputation surgeon and author of many articles on lower extremity amputations, proposed the concept that the surgeon must create a dynamic residual limb that performs as a motor and sensory end organ. Burgess suggested that the residuum functioned as a foot-like end organ and the prosthesis acted like a shoe on the foot.

Amputations should be regarded as both life-saving and function-restoring procedures that allow the patient to once again become more comfortable and return to a productive life.

References

Coleman WC, Brand PW. The diabetic foot. In Porte DJ, Sherwin RS, Eds., *Ellenberg & Rifkin's Diabetes Mellitus*, 6th ed., Stamford, CT: Appleton & Lange, 2002.

Heck RK, Carnesale PG. General Principles of Amputations. In Canale ST, Daugherty K, Jones L, Eds., *Campbell's Operative Orthopedics*, 10th ed., Vol. 1. St. Louis, MO: CV Mosby. 2003.

Levin ME, Sicard GA, Rubin BG. Peripheral vascular disease in the diabetic patient. In Porte D, Sherwin RS, Baron A, Eds., *Ellenberg & Rifkin's Diabetes Mellitus*, 5th ed., New York: McGraw-Hill Professional, 1997.

McCollough NC. Complications of Amputation Surgery. In Epps Jr C, Ed., *Complications in Orthopedic Surgery.* Philadelphia: JB Lippincott, 1986.

Pinzur MS, Stuck RM, Sage R, Hunt N, Rabinovich Z. Syme's ankle disarticulation in patients with diabetes, *J Bone Joint Surg* 85A:1667–1672, 2003.

Tooms R. Amputation of the lower extremity. In Canale ST, Daugherty K, Jones L, Eds., *Campbell's Operative Orthopedics*, 7th ed., Vol. 1. St. Louis, MO: CV Mosby, 1987.

5

The Use of Hyperbaric Oxygen in the Diabetic and Diabetic Amputees

Dennis E. Weiland, MD, FACS

History of Hyperbaric Oxygen Therapy

Hyperbaric oxygen therapy (HBOT) has been used for over a century in the treatment of various medical conditions. The first notable effort was by a French surgeon named Fontaine who built a mobile hyperbaric operating room and used nitrous oxide as an anesthetic. He reported that the cyanosis that occurred postoperatively was absent and that hernias reduced more easily. It is estimated that by using compressed air, the effective inspired oxygen level was 42% (double that of inspired air at sea level; Kindwall 1999).

In the early 20th century, Orville J. Cunningham initially treated patients with heart disease and some respiratory disorders but reported poor results. When a patient became a victim of the 1918 flu epidemic, he was placed in the chamber when respiratory complications developed and survived. Spurred by the experience, Cunningham built a chamber 88 ft. long and 10 ft. in diameter. He treated a number of diseases without scientific rationale (Jacobson, Morsch, and Rendel-Baker 1965).

In 1928, Cunningham built a three-story chamber in the form of a sphere. Pressures of three atmospheres could be achieved. It was designed as one would a luxury hotel with a smoking room at the top, plush carpeting and furniture, dining room, and individual room. He treated a number of diseases with the belief that most were caused by anaerobic organisms (they could not be cultured then).

Because of treatment failures, he was closed by the American Medical Association in 1930 (Williams 1931).

In 1878, Paul Bert produced grand mal seizures with oxygen at high pressures, demonstrating the toxicity of high concentrations of oxygen to the brain. When submarine operators had to breathe closed-circuit oxygen, a critical time of breathing needed to be developed. K. W. Donald researched this problem with Royal Navy volunteers, and helped develop safe diving charts for the U.S. Navy (Donald 1947).

During bridge construction, the footings of the bridges had to be built in caissons. They were pressurized to prevent water leaks from the surrounding river. When workers were returned to normal barometric pressures, many experienced cramps and neurological abnormalities. It produced a characteristic gait called the bends. Paul Bert had previously demonstrated that the bends were caused by nitrogen bubbles developing in the bloodstream and tissues on decompression (Kindwall 1999).

In 1889, Ernest W. Moir applied recompression to relieve decompression illness (DCI). During that time, 25% of the men employed in building the bridges died. After recompression was instituted, only 2 deaths occurred among 120 workers (Moir 1986). Today, DCI is well recognized. Divers, military personnel, and victims of surgical air emboli have hyperbaric chambers readily available to reverse DCI symptoms.

With the development of hyperbaric treatments, the Undersea Medical Society (UMS) was founded in 1967 by six U.S. Navy Diving and Submarine medical officers. In 1976, clinical hyperbaric oxygen treatments became so prevalent that the UMS became the UHMS (the Undersea Hyperbaric Medical Society). Since then, many universities have developed hyperbaric oxygen treatment programs. The UHMS also produces its own journal called *Undersea and Hyperbaric Medicine* (Kindwall 1999).

Description of Hyperbaric Chambers

Hyperbaric oxygen treatments are rendered in chambers that hold one patient (monoplace) or many patients (multiplace; Fig. 1a and 1b). Most institutions treating patients begin using monoplace chambers because they are less expensive. If the numbers of patients increase then institutions will add more chambers or add a multiplace chamber. The advantages and disadvantages of each are listed in Table 1.

In our growing population (both in numbers and patients' size), the advantage of a multiplace chamber cannot be overemphasized. The monoplace chamber's

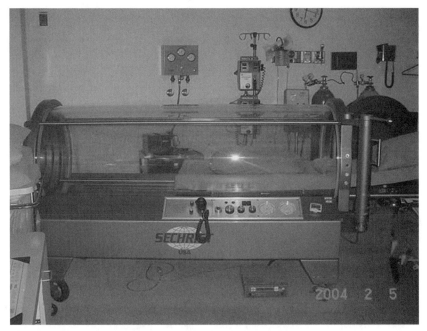

a)

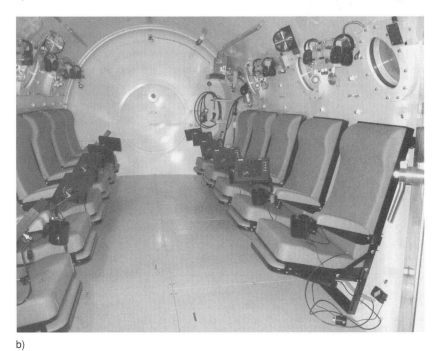

b)

Figure 1 Hyperbaric oxygen chambers. a: monoplace; b: multiplace.

Table 1 Hyperbaric Chambers: Monoplace vs. Multiplace

Condition	Monoplace	Multiplace
Claustrophobia	More	Less
Initial expense	Less	More
Inside attendant	No	Yes
Fire danger	More	Yes
Attendant procedures	No	Yes
Weight & size limit	Yes	No

small size limits the size of the patient who receives hyperbaric oxygen. Many patients with claustrophobia will not tolerate the narrow environment mandated by the small chamber size. The multiplace chamber usually eliminates both of these problems. Figure 1 shows pictures of the monoplace and multiplace chambers.

HBOTs consist of placing patients in a chamber, then pressurizing them to between 2 atmospheres absolute (2 ATA) and 3 atmospheres absolute (3 ATA). The monoplace is pressurized with 100% oxygen and the multiplace is pressurized with air, and the patient breathes 100% oxygen through a hood or mask. Treatments usually last 2 hours and continue daily for 20–30 days. A hood and mask are shown in Fig. 2a and 2b.

HBOT costs to the patient range between $150 and $900 for each treatment. The charge depends on the services offered. For example, the purchase price of multiplace chambers is 5–10 times that of a monoplace chamber. The overhead costs are greater and must be compensated by the fees charged. The number of attending personnel and the diseases treated also affect the charge. Potential

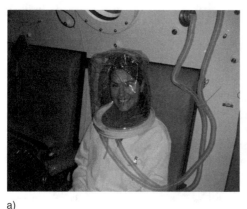
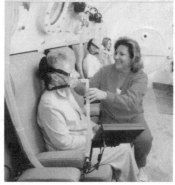

a) b)

Figure 2 Multiplace breathing equipment. a: hood; b: mask.

HBOT patients should search for the HBOT facility that meets both their medical and financial needs.

Adverse Events Using Hyperbaric Oxygen

There is one absolute contraindication to HBOT: an untreated pneumothorax. Some authorities feel that the concomitant treatment with the anticancer agents bleomycin, adriamycin, and cisplatin are also absolute contraindications. In all of these contraindications, fatal lung problems can develop with HBOT (Upton et al. 1986; Comis 1992).

Two major complications are also associated with HBOT. These include seizures from oxygen toxicity and middle ear inflammation or hemorrhage from unequalized pressure on the eardrum. Stopping the oxygen treatment and quickly reducing the pressure usually eliminates the seizure. Benzodiazepines (e.g., diazepam) are usually given for future HBOT. Middle ear problems are treated by topical or systemic decongestants (e.g., oxymetazoline or pseudoephedrine), or if severe, small tubes are placed in the eardrum to equalize pressure. Fever raises the possibility of seizures and most HBOT centers do not treat patients with a fever greater than 101 degrees unless it is an emergency.

Other minor complications from HBOT include temporary worsening of shortsightedness (myopia), "popping" of the ears, sweating, anxiety (claustrophobia), hearing impairment, and sinusitis.

Medicare Indications for Hyperbaric Oxygen

Medicare has authorized payment for diabetic wounds and associated complications. These are included in Table 2. Medicare contracts with organizations to administer hyperbaric payments to hospitals and doctors using the codes seen in Table 2. The basic payment rules are derived from the 35-10 Medicare guidelines (Centers for Medicare and Medicaid Services 2006). It is imperative that any health care organization review these regional rules before developing a hyperbaric oxygen program or they may not be paid for their services. Most insurance companies give prior payment authorization before permitting treatments. Medicare, however, is different because they review the patient's treatment after it is given. If they deem the treatment was not indicated by the regional guidelines, payment is denied. Therefore, it is very important that details of the diabetic's ulcer be documented in the consultation or the history and physical, otherwise a denial from Medicare will be sent, and the health care organization has to accept the loss. There are appeal procedures for the health care organization and if documentation is found that justifies HBOT, an appeal should be filed.

Table 2 Complicating Conditions for Which Medicare Will Approve Payment for HBOT

Condition	ICD-9 Code	Comments
Nonhealing diabetic wound	250.7( )	No progression of healing foot >30 days, Wagner grade ≥3, documented progression of healing within 30 days of HBOT
Progressive necrotizing infections	728.86	Necrotizing fasciitis, "flesh eating infections," Meleney's ulcer, Fournier's gangrene
Chronic refractory osteomyelitis	731.10, 730.19	Must be present for 6 mo. and refractory to conventional treatment
Preservation of skin grafts/flaps	996.52	Failed flaps and skin grafts, does not include skin substitutes
Acute peripheral arterial insufficiency	444.21, 444.22, 444.81	Thrombosis or embolus to a peripheral artery
Gas gangrene	040.0	Clostridial myonecrosis

Most of the guidelines for diabetic complications are relatively easy to document because they are emergencies. However, the diabetic ulcer without any serious complications becomes more difficult. Medicare's 35-10 guidelines (Table 2) for diabetic ulcerations must include the following:

1. The ulcer must be present for more than 30 days.
2. Conventional diabetic ulcer treatment must have been given for that 30-day period.
3. No progress in the ulcer's treatment must be documented.
4. The ulcer must be a Wagner's grade 3 or greater.
5. The ulcer must show improvement within 30 days after HBOT.

Because scaling the ulcer with a Wagner's scale is necessary, the definitions in the Wagner's scale are important to know and are seen in Table 3.

It is evident that advanced diabetic ulcerations are required before HBOTs are justified. It is also important to emphasize that HBOT is adjunctive to good diabetic wound care. Documentation of the improvement or regression of the ulcers(s) is essential.

Table 3 Wagner's Diabetic Ulcer Scale

Wagner's grade	Description
0	Pre-ulcerative lesions
1	Superficial ulcer (skin and subcutaneous tissue)
2	Ulcer involves fascia, tendon, joint, or ligament; no abscess or osteomyelitis
3	Deep ulcer with abscess or osteomyelitis
4	Gangrene of a portion of the foot
5	Extensive gangrene of the foot

In selecting a suitable patient, the patient and wound(s) need a thorough evaluation. The patient may have many systemic diseases contributing to the poor healing process. These include uncontrolled diabetes, heart failure, osteomyelitis, malnutrition, chemotherapy, and steroid use. The wound may be infected or contain necrotic debris. These must be corrected before the wound will heal.

Transcutaneous Oxygen Measurements

Nonhealing wounds characteristically have low oxygen levels (hypoxic). Hypoxia results from chronic scar alone or may be preceded by vascular disease, edema, or both. Large and small arteries may be narrowed or obstructed in diabetics, rendering the tissues hypoxic. An oxygen level of 30–40 mm Hg is needed to promote healing. Unless more oxygen is supplied to the wound by revascularization or by hyperbaric oxygen, the wound will not heal. Hence, it is very important to assess the wound oxygen levels. This is easily done by the use of transcutaneous oxygen measurements (TCOMs) (Figs. 3 and 4).

TCOMs are performed by placing small transducer suction cups on viable skin near the area of concern (Figure 4). The cups are heated, dilating the vessels in the skin, to allow the diffusion of oxygen (Sheffield 1988). Transducers then measure the diffused oxygen from the capillaries. The measured oxygen levels provide a simple, noninvasive, and reliable assessment of perfusion and oxygenation (Matos and Nunez 1994). Measuring TCOMs while breathing 100% oxygen helps select patients that might benefit from HBOT therapy (Brakora and Sheffield 1995; Mathieu et al. 1998).

In examining the diabetic data, the seriousness of a diabetic foot ulcer must be understood. For example, the annual incidence of foot ulcers in diabetics is estimated to be between 2.5% and 10% and the annual incidence of amputation is 0.25%–1.8% (Veves et al. 1992; Lee et al. 1993). Moreover, the relapse rate for recurrent foot ulcers is 66% over five years. In total, 12% of diabetics with foot

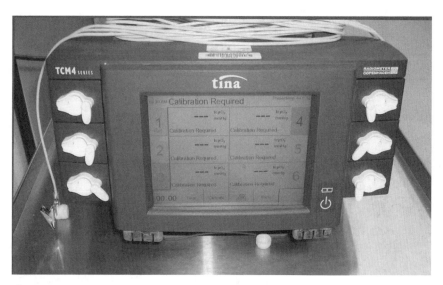

Figure 3 Transcutaneous oxygen measurement (TCOM) equipment. (Photograph is used with permission from Radiometer Medical A/S.)

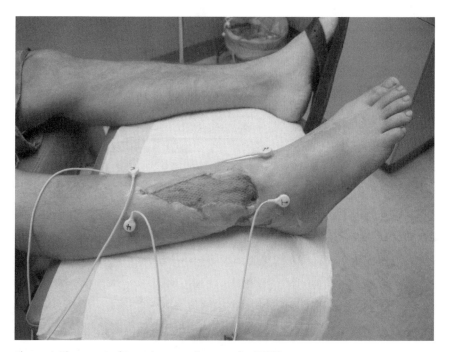

Figure 4 Placement of transducer suction cups for TCOM.

ulcers progress to lower extremity amputation (Apelqvist, Larsson, and Agardh 1993). Fife et al. (2002) analyzed 1,144 patients with TCOMs at room air, 100% oxygen, and inside the hyperbaric chamber. TCOMs on room air showed little statistical relationship predicting benefit of HBOT. TCOMs after breathing 100% oxygen showed a 68% reliability in predicting benefit. The single best predictor was oxygen levels of more than 200 mm Hg. This value predicted that 74% of patients with values higher than 200 mm Hg would benefit from HBOT (Fife et al. 2002).

TCOM readings are important in predicting a successful amputation as well. Zgonis et al. showed that a TCOM greater than 29 mm Hg was needed to have a successful partial foot amputation (Zgonis et al. 2005). Successful treatment took 44 days and 20 HBOTs while unsuccessful treatments took 216 days and 16 HBOTs (Zgonis et al. 2005).

If the amputation fails, TCOMs may be used to determine if HBOT would be useful in preserving the flap created by the amputation (a failed flap is a Medicare criterion for HBOT). If TCOM measurements are more than 200 mm Hg in the hyperbaric chamber, HBOT will be beneficial (Strauss, Breedlove, and Hart 1997).

Data Supporting the Use of Hyperbaric Oxygen in Diabetic Ulcerations

The Cochrane Collaboration is an organization that reviews medical literature using evidence-based methods to determine if medical treatments produce a significant effect on the quality of life. In the case of HBOT for diabetic ulcers, 4 randomized trials (147 patients) showed that there was a major reduction in major amputations when HBOT was used (Kranke, Bennett, Roeckl-Wiedmann, and Debus 2005). Healing rates also showed a significant improvement after one year in patients treated with HBOT.

Strauss reported his review of 12 reports showing that healing rates of diabetic foot wounds improved from 48%–76% and amputation rates decreased from 45%–19% when HBOT was used as an adjunct to conventional diabetic foot ulcer therapy (Strauss 2005). Further analysis showed remarkably similar results regardless of whether they were randomized, head-to-head, prospective, or retrospective. Once the wound is healed, the metabolic requirements are much less and should remain healed unless more trauma or vascular disease develops (Strauss 2001).

Many diabetic patients harm themselves by smoking, not following foot protocols to keep their feet from being damaged, and not keeping their diabetes under control. Otto et al. retrospectively reviewed 1,006 patients who had received

HBOTs for diabetic wounds. A smoking history was documented in 469 (47%) (Otto, Buyukcakir, and Fife 2000). Complete data were available on 180 patients. Analysis showed that patients with fewer than 10 pack-years (number of packs of cigarettes smoked per day times the number of years smoked) were not statistically different from nonsmokers. However, those patients with more than 10 pack-years required a significant increase in HBOTs (8–14 more treatments). This translates to an increase in cost of $4,000–$7,000 and an estimated $22–$37 million annually for the United States. Results show that patients who smoke are commonly found to have reduced TCOMs for 30–60 minutes following a cigarette.

Concomitant Use of HBOT and Other Diabetic Treatments

It is essential that the diabetic wound receive conventional therapy. This includes debridement, appropriate systemic and topical antibiotics (based on culture and sensitivities), proper diabetic control (HbA1C <7), and becaplermin (Regranex). Unless the wound has received these therapies, wound healing will be delayed or will not occur.

Becaplermin is a unique product. It is platelet-derived growth factor (PDGF) produced by bacteria that have been genetically engineered to produce PDGF. Placing this product in the wound has shown to accelerate the healing of many diabetic ulcerations (Smiell et al. 1999). However, some of these diabetic wounds fail to respond to becaplermin. The reason for this is obscure, but Boykin feels that some diabetic wounds produce insufficient nitric oxide (NO). Because NO is a naturally occurring vasodilator, a deficiency would make a wound ischemic and consequently slow healing (Boykin 2000). It is well known that when HBOT increases wound oxygen tensions (hyperoxia), there is an increase in wound granulation tissue formation with acceleration in wound contraction and secondary wound closure. Histologic studies show an increase in neovascularization of ischemic wounds. These new blood vessels appear to be permanent, thereby maintaining the structure of skin covering the previous wound. HBOT may mediate NO production as oxygen and L-arginine combine to produce NO. Because L-arginine is a naturally occurring amino acid, exogenous oxygen via HBOT might serve to produce more NO and assist in wound healing.

Topical hyperbaric oxygen (THBO) has been studied for more than 20 years. Earlier results in diabetic patients failed to show benefit. However, recent articles on the subject have suggested that some wounds benefit from THBO (Kallianinen et al. 2003). Edsberg et al. (2002) examined THBO, and THBO with electrical stimulation failed to demonstrate benefit. More data using THBO in randomized controlled trials are needed to determine if THBO is beneficial. Currently, insurance companies will not pay for these treatments.

All of these recommended treatments should be considered in diabetics with failed amputations. The comparison to a Wagner's grade 3 ulcer (tissue necrosis) is valid; therefore, HBOT should be considered and validated by Medicare and other insurance companies.

Conclusions

This chapter discussed the benefits of HBOT as an adjunct to diabetic foot ulcers, the prevention of amputations, and the complications of amputations once they occur. Currently, Medicare justifies HBOT for only advanced ulcers. If HBOT benefits advanced ulcers, then it should benefit diabetic ulcers in earlier stages before they develop into an advanced stage. Good evidence for earlier treatment must be developed before HBOT can be justified. It is hoped that readers of this chapter find themselves in a circumstance in which these study efforts can be made.

Not all diabetic patients benefit from HBOT. As reported earlier, nitric oxide production may be important. However, behavior of the diabetic with sugar control, proper hygiene, correct footwear, and care of associated diseases will ultimately influence the diabetic foot ulcer and its complications more than any HBOT protocol.

Hyperbaric oxygen therapy is in its infancy in the treatment of various other medical conditions. Many other ischemic diseases such as strokes and heart attacks show some evidence for the benefit of HBOT. However, HBOT is very expensive and unless there is more primary evidence (randomized control trials) showing benefit, the cost cannot be justified and HBOTs will not be given.

References

Apelqvist J, Larsson J, Agardh CD. Long-term prognosis for diabetic patients with foot ulcers. *J Intern Med* 233:485–491, 1993.

Boykin JV. The nitric oxide connection: Hyperbaric oxygen therapy, becaplermin, and diabetic ulcer management. *Adv Skin Wound Care* 13:169–74, 2000.

Brakora MJ, Sheffield PJ. Hyperbaric oxygen therapy for diabetic wounds. *Clin Pod Med Surg* 12:105–17, 1995.

Centers for Medicaid and Medicare Services, http://www.cms.hhs.gov, 2006.

Comis RL. Bleomycin Pulmonary Toxicity: Current Status and Future Directions. *Semin Oncol* 19(2, suppl 5) 64–70, 1992.

Donald KW. Oxygen poisoning in man. *BMJ* 2:712–717, 1947.

Edsberg LE, Brogan MS, Jaynes CD, Fries K. Topical hyperbaric oxygen and electrical stimulation: Exploring potential synergy. *Ostomy Wound Manage* 48:42–50, 2002.

Fife CE, Buyukcakir C, Otto GH, Sheffield PJ, Warriner RA, Love TL, Mader J. The predictive value of transcutaneous oxygen tension measurement in diabetic lower extremity ulcers treated with hyperbaric oxygen therapy: A retrospective analysis of 1,144 patients. *Wound Rep Regen* 10:198–207, 2002.

Jacobson JH, Morsch JCH, Rendel-Baker L. The historical perspective of hyperbaric therapy. *Ann NY Acad Sci* 117:651–670, 1965.

Kallianinen LK, Gordillo GM, Schlanger R, Sen CK. Topical oxygen as an adjunct to wound healing: A clinical case series. *Pathophysiology* 9(2):81–87, 2003.

Kindwall EP. *Hyperbaric Medical Practice*, 2nd ed. Flagstaff, AZ: Best Publishing Co., 1999.

Kranke P, Bennett, M, Roeckl-Wiedmann I, Debus S. Hyperbaric oxygen therapy for chronic wounds. *Cochrane Database Syst Rev* 20:CD004954, 2005.

Lee JS, Lu M, Lee VS, Russell D, Bahr C, Lee ET. Lower-extremity amputation: Incidence, risk factors and mortality in the Oklahoma Indian Diabetes Study. *Diabetes* 42:876–82, 1993.

Mathieu D, Neviere R, Boquillon N, et al. Adjunctive hyperbaric oxygen therapy in the treatment of foot lesion in diabetic patient: Selection of patients. In Proceedings of ECHM Consensus Conference on Hyperbaric Oxygen in the Treatment of Foot Lesions in Diabetic Patients. Wattel F, Mathier D, Eds. London, UK. 139–150, 1998.

Matos LA, Nunez AA. Enhancement of healing in selected problem wounds. In *Hyperbaric Medicine Practice*. Kindwall E. Ed. Flagstaff, AZ: Best Publishing Co., 589–612, 1994.

Moir EW. Tunnelling by compressed air. *J Soc Arts* 44:567–583, 1986.

Otto GH, Buyukcakir C, Fife CE. Effects of smoking on cost and duration of hyperbaric oxygen therapy for diabetic patients with nonhealing wounds. *Undersea Hyper Med* 27: 83–89, 2000.

Sheffield PJ. Tissue oxygen measurements. In JC David, TK Hunt, Eds., *Problem Wounds: The Role of Oxygen*. New York: Elsevier, 1988; 17–51.

Smiell JM, Wieman TJ, Steed DL, Perry BH, Sampson, AR, Schwab BH. Efficacy and safety of becaplermin in patients with nonhealing, lower extremity diabetid ulcers: A combined analysis of four randomized studies. *Wound Rep Regen* 7:335–346, 1999.

Strauss, MB. Diabetic foot and leg wounds: Principles, management, prevention. *Primary Care Rep* 7:187–198, 2001.

Strauss MB. Hyperbaric oxygen as an intervention for managing wounds hypoxia: Its role and usefulness in diabetic foot wounds. *Foot Ankle Int* 26:15–18, 2005.

Strauss MJ, Breedlove JW, Hart GB. Use of transcutaneous oxygen measurements to predict healing in foot wounds (Abstract). *Undersea Hyper Med* 24 (suppl):15, 1997.

Upton PG, Yamaguchi KT, Myers S, Kidwell TP, Anderson RJ. Effects of antioxidants and hyperbaric oxygen in ameliorating experimental doxorubicin skin toxicity in the rat. *Cancer Treatment Rep* 70:503–507, 1986.

Veves A, Murray HJ, Young MJ, Boulton AJ. The risk of foot ulceration in diabetic patients with high foot pressure: A prospective study. *Diabetologia* 35:660–663, 1992.

Williams, HS, Ed. *Book of Marvels.* New York: Funk and Wagnall, 1931.

Zgonis, T, Garbalosa JC, Burns P, Vidt L, Lowery C. A retrospective study of patients with diabetes mellitus after partial foot amputation and hyperbaric oxygen treatment. *J Foot Ankle Surg* 44:276–280, 2005.

6

Treatment of Diabetic Wounds with Negative Pressure Wound Therapy

Tom Wolvos, MD, FACS

Diabetic Wounds

Patients with diabetes are susceptible to the development of wounds, especially of their legs and feet. Factors that contribute to the development of these wounds include the neuropathy (decreased sensation) and the development of peripheral vascular disease (poor circulation) often seen in chronic diabetics. Not only are diabetics prone to the development of wounds, they also have a decreased ability to heal the wounds they develop. Unfortunately, it is common for many of these wounds to progress to the point that a major amputation is required. Treatment of diabetic wounds to get them to heal often requires multiple therapies, which may include surgery to remove any infected tissue, and appropriate antibiotics to treat an infection if present. Methods to increase the circulation to provide necessary oxygen to the area of the wound may include bypass surgery, angioplasty (opening up the arteries with balloons), and hyperbaric oxygen treatments. With the successful healing of the wound, an amputation can be avoided.

Another modality that is often used to treat wounds in diabetics is negative pressure wound therapy (NPWT; also called V.A.C.® therapy). Vacuum-Assisted Closure (V.A.C.®) therapy is used to treat a variety of wounds all over the body, in diabetics and nondiabetics alike. In diabetics, V.A.C.® therapy is most often used to treat leg and feet wounds to aid in their healing, thus preventing the need for an amputation. In some situations—even after an amputation has been done—there are problems with healing at the amputation wound site. V.A.C.® therapy may also be used in that situation to help heal the amputation site wound to prevent the need for further surgery.

The V.A.C.® System

V.A.C.® therapy using the V.A.C.® system (Vacuum-Assisted Closure, Kinetics Concepts Inc., San Antonio, TX) has been available for use in the United States for over a decade. The system is illustrated in the case study at the end of this chapter. The device uses an advanced foam dressing that is reticulated and open celled (has small holes in the foam that are connected to each other), along with a computerized pump that delivers negative pressure. The V.A.C.® dressing is usually done at the bedside and involves placing a piece of the advanced foam, which is cut to the size of the wound, directly into the wound. This is done without the need for anesthesia.

A semi-occlusive drape, sticky on one side, is placed over the foam and surrounding skin to achieve and maintain an airtight seal. Then suction tubing is placed over a hole cut in the drape allowing direct contact with the foam (Fig. 1). The other end of the tubing is attached to a computerized pump that delivers the negative pressure (Fig. 2). When the pump is turned on, negative pressure is delivered to the wound, causing the foam to contract and fluid and exudate to be removed from the wound. The fluid is collected in a disposable canister housed in the pump. The pump can be programmed to apply the suction in a continuous or intermittent fashion.

Typically, the dressing is left untouched in place with the pump on until it is time to be changed, usually every 48 hours. The system can be used in a hospital, extended care facility, or outpatient setting. Different pumps are available for use depending on the wound type and patient care setting (Fig. 2).

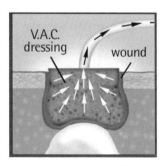

Figure 1 Illustration of the V.A.C.® foam dressing.

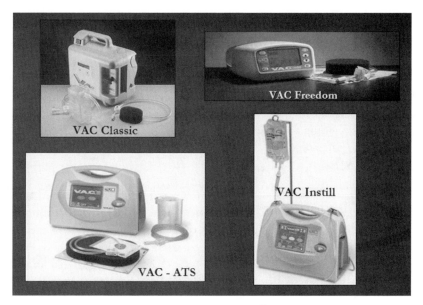

Figure 2 Pictures of the V.A.C.® pumps.

The Effects of V.A.C.® Therapy

The effects of V.A.C.® therapy on wounds have been studied (Morykwas and Argenta 1997). Negative pressure wound therapy has been shown to decrease the number of bacteria in wounds, meaning the number of bacteria fall so that the wound is no longer classified as being clinically infected. The blood flow to the wound with V.A.C.® therapy has been shown to be increased fourfold, which results in more oxygen being delivered to the wound and aiding healing. Also, the amount of granulation tissue (desirable healing tissue rich with circulation) was shown to increase by more than 60% with V.A.C.® therapy compared to the accepted standard wet-to-moist wound dressing. V.A.C.® therapy helps remove swelling or edema in the area of the wound. V.A.C.® therapy also may remove some factors in the blood and tissue that inhibit wound healing while attracting other factors that may stimulate the wound to heal (Banwell et al. 1999).

Scientists have conducted research studies to better understand how V.A.C.® therapy promotes wound healing. Computer models have demonstrated the concept that the negative pressure causes individual cells in the wound to be stretched and partially sucked into the open spaces in the foam. This stretching and straining of the cells stimulates these cells to divide, increasing the number of cells in the wound, and helps fill the wound with more desirable healing tissue (cells), which results in wound healing (Saxea 2004).

V.A.C.® Therapy and Hyperbaric Oxygen Treatments

V.A.C.® therapy can be used in conjunction with other treatment modalities such as hyperbaric oxygen therapy (HBOT). During HBOT, the V.A.C.® dressing is left in place but the tubing is disconnected from the pump. At the end of the hyperbaric treatment, the patient's V.A.C.® tubing is reattached and the V.A.C.® pump is turned back on.

The V.A.C.® Instill™ System

In the hospital setting, a modification of the V.A.C.® system—the V.A.C.® Instill™—is available to allow intermittent wound irrigations to be combined with negative pressure wound therapy (Wolvos 2004). The Instill™ system is used when traditional V.A.C.® therapy does not achieve the desired effects or it may be utilized early in a serious wound, which without aggressive care, is likely to lead to an amputation. Antiseptic solutions such as Dermacyn® (Oculus Innovative Sciences, Petaluma, CA) have been successfully used with this system (Wolvos 2006). The V.A.C.® Instill™ system is also an effective way to intermittently deliver local anesthetics to painful wounds.

Side Effects and Dressing Issues with V.A.C.® Therapy

Issues that can occur during V.A.C.® therapy include pain, bleeding, and difficulty in maintaining an airtight seal, causing the pump to function improperly. It is unusual for patients to experience significant pain while the V.A.C.® is in place and the negative pressure is being applied. Occasionally, discomfort may be noticed at V.A.C.® dressing changes. This discomfort at V.A.C.® dressing changes can be relieved by giving pain medication prior to dressing changes or, in more severe cases, by placing an anesthetics solution into the foam immediately prior to the dressing changes.

V.A.C.® therapy stimulates the formation of the desirable healing tissue, which has a rich blood supply that may bleed, in the wound. With the V.A.C.® therapy system in place, if there is noticeable or continued bleeding from the wound (such as blood in the tubing or accumulating in the canister), the patient will need to quickly inform his or her health care professionals and be evaluated.

Some wounds, due to their location, can make it difficult to maintain an airtight seal. The pump will not function properly and an alarm will sound if there is an air leak. An air leak is not dangerous but does require evaluation and treatment.

It is unusual but if the patient experiences a skin reaction to the adhesive drape, the therapy will usually need to be stopped.

Stopping V.A.C.® Therapy

V.A.C.® therapy is discontinued when the desired goal is met. The goal may be complete or near complete healing of the wound, getting the wound to the point where a skin graft or flap may be done, or healing the wound to a point where only traditional moist dressing changes are required to finish the healing process. It may require several weeks and occasionally months of V.A.C.® therapy to achieve the desired goal. V.A.C.® therapy will also be stopped in the less common situation where the wound does not appear to be improving.

Studies of the Effectiveness of V.A.C.® Therapy in Diabetic Patients

Negative pressure wound therapy seems to be a safe and effective treatment for complex diabetic wounds. The guidelines for use of V.A.C.® therapy in diabetic foot wounds have been published (Armstrong 2004). In a randomized study of diabetic patients, it was concluded that V.A.C.® therapy could lead to a higher proportion of healed wounds, faster healing rates, and potentially fewer amputations (Armstrong and Lavery 2005).

Negative pressure therapy compared to wet-to-moist dressing changes in the treatment of diabetic wounds with significant soft tissue defects has also been studied. It was concluded that V.A.C.® therapy may lead to fewer postoperative complications, the need for fewer future surgeries, and fewer readmissions to the hospital.

Summary

V.A.C.® therapy has been used for over a decade to treat the wounds often seen in diabetics. It can be used in combination with other treatment modalities. The positive effects that may be seen in a wound being treated with V.A.C.® therapy include a decrease in the number of bacteria in the wound, increased circulation to the wound, and an increase in the amount of the desirable healing (granulation) tissue seen in the wound. This may result in a higher proportion of healed wounds with fewer amputations.

The mechanism of action of V.A.C.® therapy continues to be better understood. Many studies have been published in the medical literature showing the

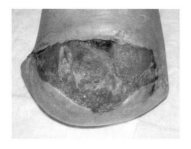

Figure 3a Open below-knee amputation wound after patient fell on his incision.

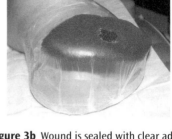

Figure 3b Wound is sealed with clear adhesive drape, making the wound airtight. A hole was cut in the drape for the suction tubing.

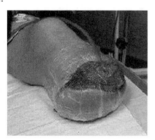

Figure 3c Suction tubing is placed over the foam.

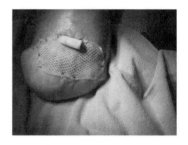

Figure 3d Tubing is attached to a suction pump.

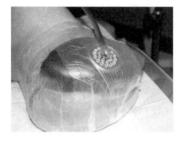

Figure 3e After suction is applied, the V.A.C.® foam collapses.

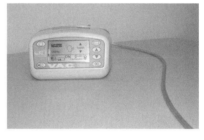

Figure 3f A partial-thickness skin graft is placed on the wound.

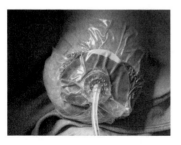

Figure 3g The skin graft is secured with the V.A.C.® system.

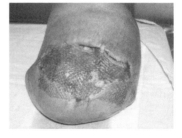

Figure 3h First dressing change occurs five days later (V.A.C.® therapy is stopped at this time).

effectiveness and safety of the V.A.C.® therapy system in the treatment of diabetic wounds.

Case Study Demonstrating V.A.C.® Dressing Changes

The patient in this case was a 45-year-old diabetic male who underwent a below-knee amputation due to a progressive uncontrolled infection of his foot. He fell on the amputation incision and the wound opened up. V.A.C.® therapy was used to prepare the wound for a skin graft and then used to hold the skin graft in place. Following skin grafting, his wound went on to complete healing (Fig. 3a–h).

References

Armstrong D, Lavery A. Negative pressure wound therapy after partial diabetic foot amputation: A multicentre, randomized controlled trial. *Lancet* 366:1704–1710, 2005.

Armstrong DG, Attinger CE, Boulton AJ, Frykberg RG, Kirsner RS, Lavery LA, Mills JL. Guidelines regarding negative pressure wound therapy (NPWT) in the diabetic foot: Results of the Tucson Expert Consensus Conference (TECC) on VAC Therapy. *Ostomy Wound Manage* 50(4 suppl B):3S–27S, 2004.

Banwell PE, Morykwas MJ, Jennings DA, McGrouther DA, Argenta LC. Application of topical subatmospheric pressure modulates inflammatory cell extravasation in experimental partial thickness injury. *Wound Rep Regen* 7:A287, 1999.

Morykwas MJ, Argenta LC. Vacuum-assisted closure: A new method for wound control and treatment: Clinical experience. *Ann Plas Surg* 38:563–76, 1997.

Page J. Retrospective analysis of negative pressure wound therapy in open foot wounds with significant soft tissue defects. *Adv Skin Wound Care* 17:354–364, 2004.

Saxea V. Vacuum-assisted closure: Microdeformations of wound and cell proliferation. *PRS* 114:1086–1096, 2004.

Wolvos T. Wound instillation: The next step in negative pressure wound therapy. Lessons learned from initial experiences. *Ostomy Wound Manage* 50:56–66, 2004.

Wolvos T. The role of super-oxidized water in advanced wound care. *Wounds* 18(1 suppl):11S–13S, 2006.

7

Getting Ready

Douglas Van Atta, CPO

Introduction

The chapter begins with general comments regarding the early role of the prosthetist and touches on the holistic impact of an amputation. Teamwork with physical therapy and the need to protect the contralateral limb are topics that lead to a review of various protocols and devices used for pre- and post-amputation care. The conclusion reinforces the basic concepts and emphasizes the importance of the early involvement of the prosthetist as part of the team.

The Power of Information

The prosthetist and prosthetic facility should be considered a resource for patients, concerned and involved family and friends, as well as other allied health professionals seeking information. The first step in regaining ambulatory function and improving a person's quality of life may be the decision to undergo an amputation. The decision for an amputation is most often very straightforward; the amputation is required as part of a life-saving strategy. However, the decision is sometimes not straightforward and may involve a struggle in reaching that conclusion. The prosthetist can be one of many resources available for the patient (see Resources and Suggested Readings).

Regardless as to how the decision to undergo an amputation is developed, the early involvement of a prosthestist is beneficial to the patient and maximizes the prosthetist's potential to have a constructive, positive impact while helping to achieve the best possible outcome. The involvement can begin preoperatively for many patients as they seek information and/or consider a decision for amputation. However, every patient should have a physician-requested prosthetic consultation as soon postoperatively as medically appropriate.

Patients and families need information as part of their recovery and rehabilitation process. The patient who may not be a candidate for a prosthesis will still benefit from a prosthetic consultation. The patient who is a candidate for a prosthesis, or who is considering the option, should be visited by a prosthetist in the acute care hospital setting even if no prosthetic procedures are utilized (Droste 1998). The lines of communication need to be opened, information needs to be shared, a relationship needs to begin, and a continuum of care should proceed with the outcome in mind.

Holistic Healing

Fear and anxiety are natural feelings for both patients and families. These feelings will mix with other traditional reactions such as sadness, anger, and eventually acceptance as the patient emotionally recovers. Several books (Madruga 1979; Riley 2005; Winchell 1995) deal with these aspects of an amputation and emphasize the fact that an amputation affects not only patients' physical reality but also their mental, emotional, and spiritual realities as well. Questions ranging from what happened to the amputated anatomy, through how to formulate a plan, to what the future holds need to be addressed in a timeframe sensitive to the patient's readiness and interest. The prosthetist's early interaction can often help move this part of recovery forward. The provision of basic facts can have a significant influence on recovery.

The patient needs to hear from the prosthetist that using a prosthesis does not involve pain and the very tender distal aspect of the residual limb is typically not going to accept weight bearing in the prosthetic design. Sores, blisters, and callous formation are inappropriate. The care of the residual limb will entail a moisturizing program and the skin should remain soft, supple, and healthy. The patient, especially a diabetic whose protective sensation is usually compromised, needs to recognize the importance of skin care and inspection. Nightly application of lanolin-based lotion after normal washing with soap and water will be the routine. Patients need to hear that they can successfully regain ambulatory function and a normal life. In addition to a prosthetic consultation, national amputee groups are active and many communities have local support groups (Kelley 2005; see Resources and Suggested Readings) and offer peer counseling for new amputees. Information is empowering and will help with the holistic healing process.

The guidance and/or involvement of a physical therapist should be a central part of any preprosthetic strategy. The physical therapy program will focus on range of motion and strengthening. Patient compliance on a daily basis is crucial because the patient is the most important variable in achieving a successful outcome. The prosthetic perspective may diverge slightly from a classic physical therapy program. The prosthetist wants strength through the full range of motion but typically is not a proponent for long-distance hopping with a walker or crutches. Functional skills such as sit-to-stand activities and transfer techniques that minimize shear forces on the remaining foot are a priority. The remaining foot needs to be protected as part of the preprosthetic program. The use of a custom insert and appropriate footwear coupled with physical therapy that minimizes mechanical stress on the remaining foot is vital. Hopefully, the contralateral foot can be preserved as part of the more functional lower extremity.

Prosthetic Options

The technical and device options with the associated theories will be presented from the very basic, through the somewhat routine, to the more complex. The prosthetic protocols in consultation with the prosthetist are physician-directed first by the surgeon and later by a physiatrist (physical medicine and rehabilitation specialist), or another managing physician. Initially, a postsurgical dressing is applied by the surgeon in the operating room. It will be soft and sterile in nature and combine nonadherent products, absorbent pads, and a gauze wrap. The surgical dressing will be changed by the surgeon unless otherwise directed. It is at this point that a strategic path of management begins based on discussion and consideration of the options.

The routine covering applied over the surgical dressing is an elastic wrap. The main goal of this wrap is to provide compression and control edema. Additionally, a properly applied figure-eight wrap that is reapplied multiple times a day will mechanically support the wound, begin the shaping process of the residual limb, and offer some protection against bumping. There are many options for further protection that will be presented, but even something as simple as a knee immobilizer is advisable. An immobilizer, sometimes equipped with a distal cap

(Fig. 1), will promote knee extension, provide another layer of protection for the residual limb, and improve comfort for the patient by means of the additional support. Healing is always the priority. Therefore, compression and protection are the basic principles in the preprosthetic phase.

Rigid Dressings

The next categories of auxiliary coverings for the healing residual limb are rigid dressings (Kostuik 1981). The fundamental theories involved are based on nonelastic edema control, tissue/joint immobilization, and protection from blunt blow irritations and injuries. This concept relies on providing a maximally protected environment for the healing residual limb where postoperative edema is not permitted to exert a stretching and separating effect on the suture site. This type of dressing may be either removable or nonremovable.

Nonremovable Rigid Dressings

The nonremovable rigid (Fig. 2) dressing is typically applied by the prosthestist in the operating room as soon as the surgeon has applied the sterile surgical dressing. It is essentially a cast that utilizes some basic prosthetic principles in its application and minimizes excessive padding. It can be plaster, fiberglass, or a combination. An ancillary waist belt is usually provided to help keep the cast suspended and in place, especially during standing and transfer activities. The prosthetist needs to be closely involved in managing this dressing and any slippage of the cast should be immediately reported.

Specific protocols in using a nonremovable rigid dressing are directed by the surgeon. Undisturbed edema control for the first 48–72 hours is vital, but many surgeons prefer this type of dressing to remain in place between 10 and 21 days if cast suspension remains secure and there are no systemic indications that the wound needs attention. The patient frequently reports a vice-like feeling from the cast during the initial postoperative period and for up to a week. The patient should be encouraged to perceive this as a positive effect of the cast as the residual limb is trying to become engorged but the cast is preventing this engorgement and the associated negative consequences for wound healing.

Removable Rigid Dressings

Removable rigid dressings (Wu et al. 1979) can be directly fabricated on the patient (Fig. 3) or be custom fabricated to a model of the patient's residual limb

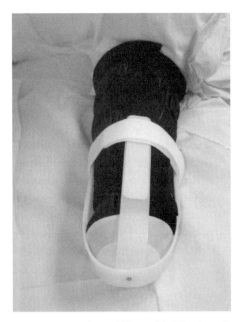

Figure 1 Knee immobilizer with "distal cap."

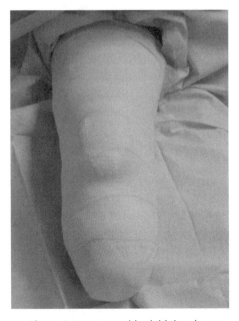

Figure 2 Nonremovable rigid dressing.

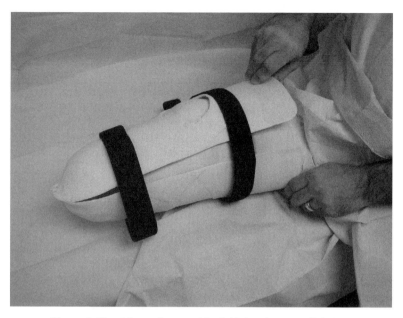

Figure 3 Direct formed removable rigid dressing—medial view.

(Fig. 4). Also, prefabricated systems are commercially available (Figs. 5 and 6). The rigid dressing should be removed as directed by a strategic protocol and only by the physician, prosthetist, or other clearly designated team member such as a nurse or physical therapist. This type of system requires very close management and education, from the prosthetist to the caregivers and patient, as the rigid dressing will be removed and reapplied. This obviously creates more risk for the distal amputation wound and great care is required as any volume changes in the residual limb need to be accommodated in the reapplication of the dressing. The involvement of a prosthetist is important and all the team members need to be educated in the utilization of this dressing.

The advantages of this approach are many but the risk and management requirements need to be acknowledged. This approach again offers rigid containment and protection for the residual limb. The removal provides for visual inspection of the wound, allows for the introduction of an elastic shrinker (tubular or sock design) (Fig. 7), and patient education regarding the concept of sock management can begin as the volume of the residual limb decreases. The desensitization of the residual limb can begin along with a range-of-motion program. Silicone or urethane liners may also be introduced with physician approval. The advantages of a removable rigid dressing are significant but the healing of the residual limb wound must not be jeopardized.

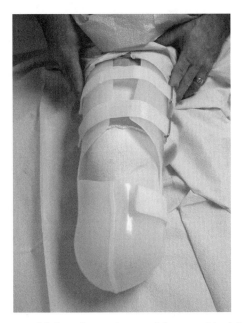

Figure 4 Custom fabricated to patient model, removable rigid dressing.

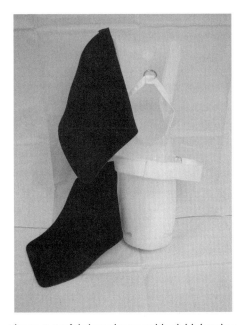

Figure 5 Prefabricated removable rigid dressing.

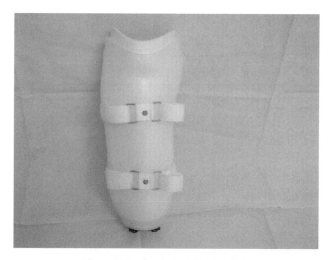

Figure 6 Prefabricated rigid socket.

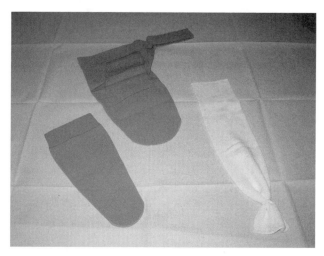

Figure 7 Transfemoral shrinker with waist belt, sock design, and tubular design transtibial shrinkers.

Immediate Postoperative Prosthesis

The last approach to be presented is that of the immediate postoperative prosthesis (IPOP) (Burgess, Romano, and Zettl 1969) and the early fitted prosthesis (Fig. 8). Both of these systems can be removable or nonremovable. Both can be directly fabricated to the patient, may be custom fabricated, or may be a commercially available system (Fig. 9). These systems are designed for partial weight

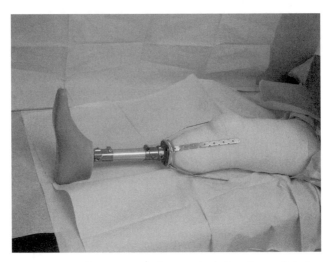

Figure 8 Immediate postoperative prosthesis (IPOP)—medial view.

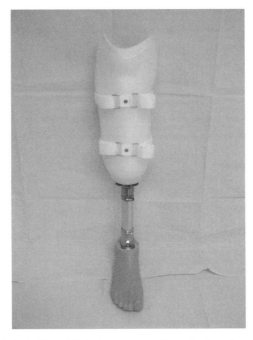

Figure 9 Early fit prefabricated socket and prosthetic pylon and foot.

bearing only. They do allow the opportunity for the patient to begin to establish balance using the residual limb and to begin some carefully supervised bipedal ambulation. However, the very real mechanical stresses, both pressure and shear, create a potentially dangerous situation for the residual limb. The prosthetist and physical therapist need to work closely together in a rehabilitation setting to increase the likelihood of success with this approach. A very mindful and cautious physical therapy program needs to follow well-established strategic protocols that emphasize specific limitations on weight bearing and activity.

The short hospital stays and lack of insurance reimbursement for rehabilitation in today's health care environment make this a less utilized option than in the past. Additionally, the delicate nature of the diabetic patient's circulatory and neurological systems creates more issues for consideration. These issues, combined with the demands this approach places on the remaining leg, the upper extremities, and the trunk, make the IPOP procedure less attractive in the diabetic population than in the traumatic amputee situation where there is an isolated injury and all other systems are intact and healthy.

Summary

The course of treatment for a given patient may involve a combination of several options. The physician may direct a sequence of procedures such as starting with a nonremovable rigid dressing applied in the operating room. This could be followed by a joint visit in the surgeon's office with the prosthetist at two weeks postoperation. The nonremovable dressing may be removed (usually with a cast saw), half of the stitches or staples may also be removed, and a removable type of dressing might be reapplied. Other components such as shrinkers, liners, and socks can be introduced at this time.

These technical aspects of care need to be supplemented with communication and information. There are pamphlets available (e.g., Shurr 1998) that cover things such as the need for elevation, residual limb shaping and volume reduction with eventual stabilization being the goal, and the importance of range of motion. They typically include an introduction to prosthetic concepts as well. The prosthetist provides these pamphlets to the patient and discusses other valuable resources when there is interest.

To conclude, there are many options and physician-directed protocols routinely used and followed in today's environment. The preprosthetic phase should focus on healing, protection, and preparation for full weight bearing on the amputated extremity via a prosthesis. The earlier in the patient's care the patient begins rehabilitation with a prosthesis designed for full weight bearing, the better.

Generally, if all goes well, this will occur at four to six weeks postamputation. A quality preprosthetic program with the participation of a prosthetist as part of the team will maximize the potential for a timely positive outcome.

Resources

American Academy of Orthotists and Prosthetists
526 King Street, Suite 201
Alexandria, Virginia 22314
703-836-0788
www.oandp.org

American Amputee Foundation, Inc.
P.O. Box 250218
Little Rock, AZ 72225
501-666-2523
www.americanamputee.org

Amputee Coalition of America
900 E. Hill Avenue, Suite 285
Knoxville, TN 37915-2568
888-267-5669
www.amputee-coalition.org

References

Burgess, EM, Romano, RL, Zettl, JH. *The Management of Lower Extremity Amputations*, Prosthetic and Sensory Aids Service, U.S. Veterans Administration, Washington DC, Bulletin T.R. 10-6, U. S. Government Printing Office, 1969.

Droste, TM. Beyond clinical care. *O & P Almanac*, July 1998, p. 42–46.

Kelley, R. Support groups. *O & P Business News*, November 1, 2005, p. 36–40.

Kostuik, JP. *Amputation Surgery and Rehabilitation—The Toronto Experience*. New York: Churchill Livingston, Inc., 1981.

Madruga, L. *One Step at a Time: A Young Woman's Inspiring Struggle to Walk Again*. New York: McGraw-Hill Book Company, 1979.

Shurr, DG. *A Manual for Above-Knee Amputees, Muilenburg Prosthetics and Orthotics*, 5th ed. Alexandria, VA: Rehabilitation Press, 1998.

Riley, RL. *Living with a Below-Knee Amputation: A Unique Insight from a Prosthetist/Amputee*. Therofare, NJ: Slack, Inc., 2005.

Winchell, E. *Coping with Limb Loss: A Practical Guide to Living with Amputation for You and Your Family/Sound Information from an Emotional Recovery Counselor Who Has Herself Experienced Amputation.* Garden City Park, NY: Avery Publishing Group, 1995.

Wu, Y, Keagy, RD, Krick, HJ, Stratigos, JS, Betts, HB. An innovative removable rigid dressing technique for below-the-knee amputation. *J Bone Joint Surg* 61:724–729, 1979.

8

Lower Limb Amputee Rehabilitation

David P. Guy, MS, PT

Introduction

The rehabilitation program after an amputation is a multiphase process. It actually begins prior to the amputation and continues for the remainder of the patient's life. To be effective, the process must be a coordinated team activity. The team, at a minimum, includes the following: the patient, the patient's family, the primary care physician, the surgeon, the diabetes educator, the prosthetist, the physical therapist, the occupational therapist, and the health insurer. Often, a social worker and psychologist are added to the team. These team players must have a defined team plan and must communicate often and effectively. Most health insurers cover the cost of the preoperative and postoperative rehabilitation programs. However, some insurers limit the number of rehabilitation visits that a patient may have per calendar year. It is, therefore, very important for the rehabilitation provider to secure prior authorization for all potential rehabilitation services and to plan to ration these services if there is a restriction on the number of rehabilitation visits that will be funded by the insurer.

It is very important to inform the patient that not all new amputees are candidates for prostheses and that the decision whether or not to use a prosthesis is often delayed until after surgery.

What follows is a presentation of activities that must be included in any successful amputee rehabilitation program for those patients who will be prosthetic users.

Preamputation Assessment and Treatment

A thorough assessment of the patient prior to surgery is essential to facilitate the postamputation rehabilitation. The preamputation assessment includes multiple components, all of which are necessary to assure the best outcome from the amputation. The physical and occupational therapists evaluate the patient's strength in all limbs and the trunk to assure that there is adequate strength to transfer between chair, bed and commode and sufficient strength to walk with an ambulation assistive device after surgery. In most cases, the patient will need to use either crutches or a walker. Similarly, the motion available in all limbs, focusing particularly on the joints immediately proximal to the amputation site, must be evaluated. Having contractures or tightness in nonaffected joints might significantly interfere with recovery, specifically whether the patient can use a prosthesis. The patient's ability to coordinate one-, two-, and four-limb activities is also very important because the patient will require good coordination to walk after surgery both with and without the eventual prosthesis. Likewise, the patient's static and dynamic balance while sitting and standing must be assessed to assure the capacity to successfully use a prosthesis.

An analysis of superficial and deep sensation in the extremities and identification of any loss of touch sensation, proprioception, or hot/cold sensation proximal to the amputation site and in the unaffected limbs is also helpful in determining the correct rehabilitation program. Checking sensation and deep tendon reflexes in both lower extremities can also help indicate any neurological problems that may co-exist with the pathology necessitating the amputation.

Checking skin integrity—whether any wounds are present on the nonsurgical limb—will also help in the development of the appropriate rehabilitation response. Clear documentation of these wounds by type and location is essential and photographs are very helpful.

The patient's ability to ambulate and whether there is a need for an assistive device is also essential to help adequately prepare to get the patient out of bed and walking as soon as possible after surgery. Early ambulation after surgery is one of the best means to prevent complications postoperatively.

The occupational therapist will spend time assessing the patient's relative independence in typical activities of daily living with the plan to assure that the patient maintains or improves in independent activity after surgery. An important component of the independence assessment is to determine the patient's understanding and use of techniques for work simplification and energy conservation. Work simplification refers to the process of adapting activities to enhance independence. For example, placing most commonly used kitchen items at or near waist height lessens the need to bend and lift, thereby decreasing the risk for falls or other injuries. Energy conservation is closely allied to work simplification, and, as it implies, it is the process of determining the most efficient way to complete tasks. Both energy conservation and work simplification are essential because the use of a prosthesis is a task requiring great amounts of energy. Another part of the analysis of the patient's abilities to perform activities of daily living is to assess the home environment to assure that the home is conducive to retaining or improving the patient's abilities. The assessing therapist will provide a list of suggested home modifications and/or additions. Finally, the patient's cognition and ability to cooperate with treatment will be assessed to assure that the patient will be able to fully participate in the rehabilitation program.

Subsequent to this assessment, if time is available prior to surgery, the therapists will provide a presurgical treatment program to lessen any deficits identified in the assessment. There may be a need for outpatient or home-health-based professional care if the patient is not hospitalized. If so, the therapists will contact the attending physician to acquire the needed prescriptions for preoperative care and then secure health insurance approval.

As part of the presurgical care, whether in the hospital, in an outpatient clinic, or with a home health service, the therapists will explain the postoperative program to both the patient and the patient's family.

A presurgical and postoperative exercise program for the nonsurgical side may be required to increase the function of that extremity and to lessen the potential problems that may interfere with the surgical side rehabilitation. This program will also focus on helping maintain the viability of the nonsurgical limb if problems do exist. (See Chapter 2 on limb preservation.)

The physician and the diabetes educator should assess diabetes control and should review and update the diabetes treatment plan. Good control is essential before surgery. Hyperglycemia increases the risk of infection and increases the risk of poor wound healing. Also, the diabetes educator should inform the patient that blood glucose levels will vary with the intensity and duration of exercise. Blood glucose monitoring is important before and after exercise to determine whether there is a need to modify either diet or medication. Finally, the diabetes educator should inform the patient and the other team members to schedule exercise 1–1$\frac{1}{2}$ hours after a meal.

If possible, the patient and family might benefit from meeting an amputee patient who has concluded treatment. Much can be gained from interpatient communication.

Immediate Postsurgical Care

Many of the procedures in this section apply not only to this segment of care but also to the entire postsurgical treatment. Care typically begins the day after surgery with the physical therapist providing a series of treatments. First, range-of-motion activities to the unaffected limbs and to the residual limb are provided to maintain or increase flexibility. Preventing joint contractures is essential to assure the best possible prosthetic fitting and subsequent gait pattern. Second, the therapist will work on getting the patient up in a chair and, if possible, walking with a walker or crutches. As stated previously, getting the patient up early is one of the best means to prevent complications of surgery and anesthesia. Third, strengthening exercises for the upper extremities will be provided. Breathing exercises are also often started to prevent pulmonary problems and to help with endurance. Some therapists will also start the patient on a program to desensitize the residual limb and to prepare for prosthetic fitting. The desensitization treatment usually consists of gentle tapping on the residual limb with a folded towel. The tapping becomes more vigorous as the residual limb becomes less sensitive. The therapist will also explain about phantom limb sensations and how the desensitization program may lessen phantom limb problems.

The occupational therapist will begin to have the patient become independent as quickly as possible with self-care and assure full functional use of both upper extremities. Usually, physical and occupational therapy is provided twice daily. As the patient improves, the therapists will require more ambulation and increased self-care independence.

Also of critical importance is proper positioning of the residual limb. For the above-knee amputee, make sure that while in bed no pillows are placed under the residual limb so that the hip is bent up. Likewise, make sure that the residual limb is held in a straight-line position with the rest of the body and that the residual limb is not held out to the side. For the below-knee amputee, make sure that no pillows are placed under the knee causing the knee to be held in a bent position. If the residual limb is held in any of the previously mentioned positions, there is an increased risk that the joints will contract in a position that will interfere with prosthetic fitting. With most amputees, it is appropriate to have the patient lay on the stomach for 20 minutes twice daily. Amputee patients should limit sitting to no more than three hours daily initially. Once they stand from a seated position, the amputee should extend fully the knee and/or the hip joints to maintain full extension mobility. Please see Figs. 1a and b and 2a and b, which demonstrate the appropriate and inappropriate bed positions.

In addition to the focus on maintaining and improving joint/muscle function, the therapy team will also address cardiopulmonary and vascular concerns. Amputee rehabilitation requires good cardiopulmonary function. The amputee patient requires great stamina to walk with a prosthesis and maintain a safe gait pattern. Also, amputee rehabilitation places a great demand on residual limb and unaffected limb vascular structures. To assure sufficient cardiopulmonary

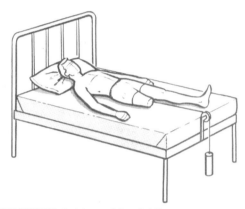

SUPINE POSITION: hips level, stump parallel to unaffected leg.

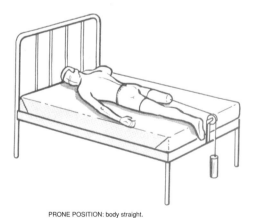

PRONE POSITION: body straight.

Figure 1a Correct positioning of an above-knee stump.

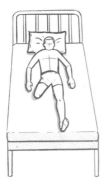

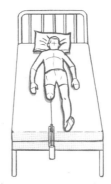

AVOID: external rotation and abduction of the stump -- conductive to undesirable contractures.

AVOID: hips uneven -- an asymmetrical position frequently occurs with fraction.

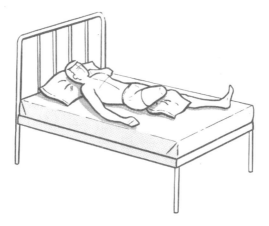

AVOID: pillow under stump -- conductive to hip flexion contracture.

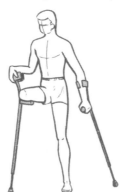

AVOID: stump resting on crutch handle -- conductive to hip flexion contracture.

Figure 1b Positions to be avoided by the above-knee amputee.

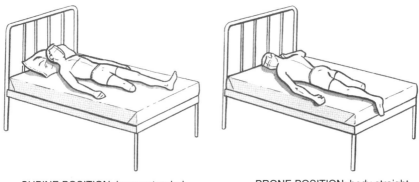

SUPINE POSITION: knee extended.

PRONE POSITION: body straight, knee extended.

Figure 2a Correct positioning of a below-knee stump.

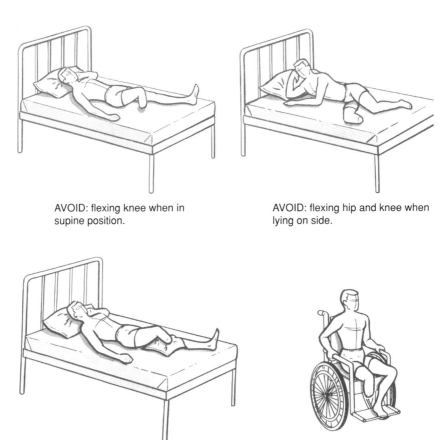

AVOID: flexing knee when in supine position.

AVOID: flexing hip and knee when lying on side.

AVOID: placing pillow under knee.

AVOID: flexing stump when sitting in wheelchair.

Figure 2b Positions to be avoided by the below-knee amputee.

capability, the therapists will provide an extensive program of endurance activities that will enhance heart–lung function. Likewise, most therapists will institute exercise programs to stimulate vascular function in the residual limb and in the unaffected limb.

Treatment will continue on a daily basis as previously mentioned with the addition of residual limb wrapping as soon as the surgeon gives approval. Figs. 3a and b illustrate diagrams of appropriate residual limb wrapping techniques.

Residual limb wrapping and the eventual use of a residual limb shrinker are essential to help control swelling and to form the limb. The residual limb wraps are usually 3- or 4-inch wide elastic bandages. These bandages need to be reapplied every two hours, as they tend to bunch up or unravel after being worn for several hours. The nursing and rehabilitation staff will check the residual limb often to assure adequate blood flow is not impeded by the wrap. The physical therapist will measure and record residual limb girth and relay these very important measures to the prosthetist. Typically, prosthetic fitting is delayed until these girth measurements stabilize and are consistent over a period of several days.

The patient and family will be taught a home program that will commence upon discharge from the hospital. Discharge criteria vary but usually include a generally stable health situation, limited wound drainage, resolution of the effects of anesthesia, and independence in ambulation and self-care.

The prosthetist will often make a visit during hospitalization to provide a residual limb shrinker sock and a residual limb protector. The prosthetist will initiate a discussion with the patient and family about prosthetic care and may take initial measurements for the first prosthesis. The therapists will often participate in this meeting and should be encouraged to do so to provide the prosthetist with information about the patient's goals and progress to this point.

Although the practice has decreased in the past decade, some physicians will request that the prosthetist provide an initial temporary prosthesis, usually made out of cast materials and a pylon with an attached prosthetic foot. If the limb has been amputated above the knee, the initial temporary prosthesis may or may not have a knee joint. This temporary prosthesis is often worn around the clock, eliminating the use of residual limb wraps or shrinkers.

Postacute Hospital Rehabilitation

Three potential environments are available to most patients on discharge from the acute-care hospital. The choice of which environment is determined by the surgeon in consultation with the rest of the rehabilitation team. The decision is

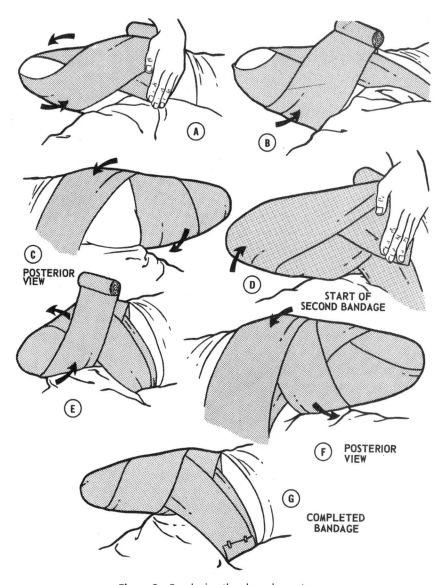

Figure 3a Bandaging the above-knee stump.

often dependent on the patient's general health, results of the in-hospital rehabilitation care, and insurance coverage.

Home health care may or may not be ordered by the physician. This service can only be ordered if the patient is and remains homebound during all care that may be provided. Homebound refers to the patient's inability to get out of the

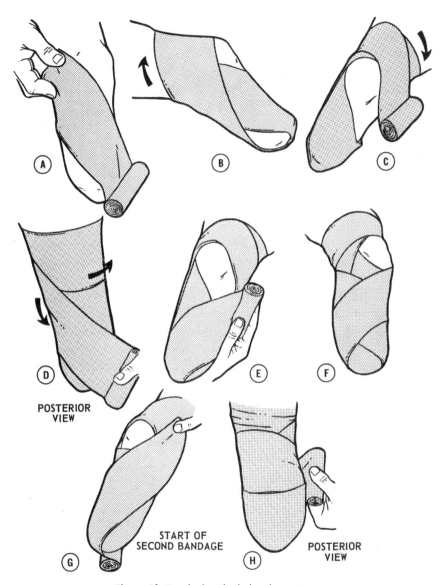

Figure 3b Bandaging the below-knee stump.

home for other than physician visits or other essential out-of-home activities. It also means that getting the patient out of the home requires great effort. If it is ordered, a home health agency will call to arrange home visits. Usually, nurses and home health aides along with therapists will be provided. The nurses will assess general health concerns and monitor the surgical wound healing. The home health aides will often assist with personal hygiene and bathing. Most insurers cover the expense for this service.

If home health care is not appropriate, continued care may be provided in an outpatient rehabilitation clinic. Most hospitals provide these services, as do many private rehabilitation facilities.

The third alternative is the rehabilitation hospital. The rehabilitation hospital provides intensive therapy and nursing care in an inpatient environment.

Regardless of the environment chosen, the therapists will continue to provide the same program as was initiated in the hospital. The program will include many exercises, several of which the amputee patient will be asked to complete outside of therapy treatment sessions (Tables 1 and 2).

The prosthetist will meet with the patient either in the home, the acute rehabilitation hospital, or the outpatient rehabilitation clinic as soon as the physicians and physical therapists agree the prosthetic fitting process may begin. The therapist, as noted previously, will make repeated measures of limb girth along with measures of strength, balance, and mobility and report these statistics to the prosthetist. During this meeting with the prosthetist, the initial prosthetic measurements may be taken and the prosthetist may begin fabrication of the prosthesis. The therapists will continue to work on improvement of all functions related to activities of daily living and assure that no avoidable problems occur. Again, as stated earlier, these avoidable problems include joint contractures, a lack of strength and/or endurance, and vascular-related problems.

Table 1 Mid-Thigh Amputation Exercises

1   Hip extension from the prone position with care that thigh is not abducted. Raising the opposite arm simultaneously prevents twisting of the body.
2   With the pelvis "squared" the thighs are adducted and internally rotated.
3   The hip is extended as the spinal column is straightened. Starting from the prone position the torso is pushed upward and back as the stump and hip are extended.
4   Lying on the side of the intact leg, the hip is flexed to stabilize the lumbar spine as the stump is extended.
5   With the torso on a table, and the intact foot on the floor, the stump is vigorously extended to increase the range of motion of the hip.
6   Resistive exercise of the hip extensors. The stump end is pushed down forcibly against a padded stool so the pelvis is lifted from the mat.
7   Resistive exercise of the hip abductors. The lateral side of the stump is pushed down forcibly against a padded stool so the pelvis is lifted from the mat.
8   Resistive exercise of the hip adductors. The medial side of the stump is pushed down forcibly against a padded stool so the pelvis is lifted from the mat.

Table 2 Below-the-Knee Amputation Exercises

1 Lying on the back, straighten the knee on the amputated side and hold straight, tightening the muscle on top of the thigh and holding it tight for a count of 10. Complete 20 repetitions.
2 Fill a pair of socks with sand and tie the ends together. Lying on the back drape the socks filled with sand over the residual limb below the knee. Keep the knee straight and lift the limb up about three inches. Complete 20 repetitions.
3 Lying on the back, push down on the entire residual limb attempting to push the residual limb into the bed/mat and hold pushing down for a count of 10. Complete 20 repetitions.
4 Lying on the side of the amputation, attempt to push the residual limb into the bed/mat holding for a count of 10. Complete 20 repetitions.
5 Place a rolled towel between the knees and squeeze the knees together, holding for a count of 10. Complete 20 repetitions.
6 Lying on the back, with both hands pull the nonamputated side knee up toward the same side shoulder while simultaneously keeping the amputated side residual limb flat against the bed/mat. Complete 5 repetitions.
7 Standing, holding onto a firm surface, move the amputated side hip backwards as far as possible without the trunk bending forward. Complete 20 repetitions.

Prosthetic Training Phase

A whole new phase begins when the prosthetist delivers the prosthesis. This initial prosthesis will not be complete. It may not have all the components of a fully completed prosthesis such as the covering of the pylon that extends from the residual limb socket to the foot. However, the initial or the preparatory prostheses will allow the patient to begin prosthetic training in earnest. The physical therapist will focus on two tasks. The first task is to teach the patient the appropriate technique in donning and removing the prosthesis and the appropriate care and cleaning of the prosthesis and the residual limb. The second task is appropriate prosthetic ambulation. The therapist will limit the time the amputee can wear the prosthesis and will gradually increase this time as the amputee demonstrates no ill effects from wearing the prosthesis and gains independence in its donning and removal. Typically, the amputee will only wear the prosthesis for two hours or less in the first week and will gradually increase wear time. The therapist will closely examine the residual limb after prosthetic use to determine if there are any problems such as swelling, persistent skin discoloration, or chaffing. The amputee needs to be educated to report any sensations of numbness, burning, or pain while wearing the prosthesis.

The amputee will be informed that the residual limb will change in size as the prosthesis is worn. This is quite normal and may require the fabrication and fitting of a new prosthetic socket.

During the ambulation training with the prosthesis, the physical therapist will perform one or more gait analyses and prosthetic checkouts. These evaluations will include an assessment of the function of the prosthesis that will assist the prosthetist in modifying the prosthesis for best fit and function. It also includes an assessment of how the amputee uses the prosthesis and what training needs should be addressed to assure appropriate prosthetic ambulation. The findings of the gait analyses and prosthetic checkouts are shared with the physicians and other members of the rehabilitation team.

Based on the gait analyses and the prosthetic checkouts, treatment will be modified to assure the best possible prosthetic system is employed and that the amputee can perform all necessary prosthetic activities. These activities include walking on level surfaces, up and down curbs, stairs and inclines, in and out of vehicles, on and off chairs and commodes, how to pick things up from the floor, correct falling techniques, and how to rise from the floor. How to get through a day with a prosthesis from brushing the teeth to having dinner at a restaurant will be explained. Also the treatment to increase strength, endurance, coordination, and balance will be determined. Generally, the amputee patient will be taught to be an effective and efficient user of both his or her physical skills and the technology fabricated in the prosthesis. As training continues, the therapist may change or eliminate the use of assistive devices. Frequently, patients begin ambulation in parallel bars, progress to a walker or crutches and, from there, to a cane. Some amputees become so proficient with their prosthesis that they learn to ambulate with no assistive device.

As the training proceeds, the prosthetist will complete the final definitive prosthesis. The entire process of rehabilitation, from the amputation to completion of training with the definitive prosthesis, can be completed in as little as several months but could take a year. The time required is dependent on multiple factors that may be evident at the outset but may not be clear until well into the prosthetic training. A comprehensive and complete initial assessment is often the critical factor in estimating the length and success of rehabilitation.

Postcare Follow-up

Once the four phases of care are complete, the patient begins the final phase of care that will continue for the rest of his or her life. The patient and family will be instructed in assessment of the residual limb and the prosthesis to gain the skills needed to identify incipient issues before they become problems. The amputee and family will also be encouraged to communicate regularly with the prosthetist and the physical therapist and to use these professionals as a resource to answer any questions. There are few inappropriate questions. As with the earlier phases of care, communication between the patient and the caregivers is essential. Likewise, the diabetes educator and primary care physician also need to gain the skills required to identify potential problems.

Of particular concern is a frequent skin check, particularly the area around the limb at the top of the prosthesis. With the above-knee amputee, the skin in the groin and the skin over the ischial tuberosity need frequent checks to assure that the skin has not been damaged. With the below-knee amputee, the skin over the head of the fibula and the distal tibia must be assessed. An easy assessment is to check the skin with the prosthesis off and determine if there is any discoloration of the skin that persists for more than 20 minutes after the prosthesis is removed. Second, check to see if the skin is either warm or cold. Extremes of either temperature can indicate developing problems. Also check to see if light touch, hot–cold, and deep pressure sensations are intact. Third, with the prosthesis on the amputee, examine the area around the top of the prosthesis to determine whether there are any skin folds over the top of the prosthesis. Finally, ask the patient whether there is any pain or burning sensation when he or she wears the prosthesis. Any changes noted in this evaluation should be reported to the prosthetist and physical therapist. The amputee needs to continue to wear the residual limb shrinker whenever the prosthesis is off. Failure to wear the shrinker may cause the residual limb to enlarge and, therefore, not fit appropriately in the prosthesis.

Continued vigilance and communication will help assure that the amputee continues to be an efficient and effective prosthesis user and to avoid unnecessary sequelae to the amputation.

Suggested Readings

Bild DE, Selby JV, Sinnock P, Browner WS, Braveman P, Showstack JA. Lower-extremity amputation in people with diabetes: Epidemiology and prevention. *Diabetes Care* 12:24–31, 1989.

Esquenazi A. Geriatric amputee rehabilitation. *Clin Geriatr Med* 9(4):731–743, 1993.

Dillingham TR. Amputee rehabilitation can improve results. *BioMech*. 1999. Available from http://www.biomech.com/db_area/archives/1999/9908oandp.45-53.bio.html. Accessed December 7, 2006.

Ham R, Regan JM, Roberts VC. Evaluation of introducing the team approach to the care of the amputee: The Dulwich study. *Prosthet Orthot Intl* 11:25–30, 1987.

Rommers GM, Vos LD, Groothoff JW, Eisma WH. Clinical rehabilitation of the amputee: A retrospective study. *Prosthet Orthot Intl* 20(2):72–78, 1996.

9

Overview of Lower Limb Prostheses

Steve McNamee, CP

Introduction

Diabetes is a disease that can lead to many bodily ailments, with one of the most visually stunning being that of limb loss. The lower extremity, being farthest from the heart and with the smallest vessels, suffers the most. When wounds do not heal, infection can spread. Tissue becomes necrotic, with amputation often the result. Although it may seem harsh, it is necessary to stop the infection from spreading even further.

Amputations most commonly occur below the knee. Blood flow typically becomes more restricted below the major calf muscles. With proper monitoring and medical oversight, clinicians must stop the progression of problems at this point. A prosthesis fit below the knee is generally well accepted and utilized by the patient and requires the least energy expenditure to use. Amputations above the knee can also be quite useful in returning patients to normal daily activity. However, they do require greater energy output and are more technical in nature because of the addition of a knee joint. Because of these facts, emphasis in this chapter will be placed on lower extremity amputation and the associated prosthetic care.

Hopefully, most diabetic patients have had care and counsel to monitor their feet. Daily examination and care for skin cracks, problem toenails, and blisters is critical. These issues certainly affect all people, but the wound care issues surrounding the diabetic make them even more significant. If amputation occurs, the same diligence is needed to ensure continuity of daily prosthetic use. Manufacturers have made efforts to address these needs by developing items that cushion, protect, and unload fragile diabetic tissue. These items will be covered later in this chapter.

In my fifteen years of experience, the majority of my patients have been diabetic. I have been honored to look after many of the Native American Indians in Arizona. It has been suggested that historically abrupt changes in diet and activity levels have led to one of the highest per capita diabetic rates in the world. Whatever the cause, diabetes results in many amputations. It is rare that I receive a new patient unfamiliar with a prosthesis, most having seen Mom, Dad, or a grandparent who used one. I note this because I think it is of significance in the high rate of success achieved with fittings.

Because of an initial background knowledge and exposure to artificial limbs, my patients seem more likely to accept and use the device with as much normalcy as can be expected. A return to daily life with little dependence on or assistance from family or friends is an expected outcome. While many of your patients may not come from this background, nor have had any exposure at all to prosthetics, or may be scared to death by the thought of losing a body part, please take heart in the following: With today's technology, an amputee has every opportunity to return to independent daily activities with minimal discomfort or problems associated with the prosthesis. While this statement may oversimplify the use of a prosthesis, I hope that those reading this book will be optimistic in any conclusions they may draw on being an amputee. Many things are involved in a prosthetic fitting. Certainly, it is not an easy process, and each patient is different and will present unique issues that influence the fitting outcome. Many options are available, however, increasing the choices for both wearer and provider.

Much emphasis should rest on the interaction between the patient and his or her prosthetist. The prosthetist should have some level of national certification, indicating an educational background in anatomy, physiology, and biomechanics. The relationship between the amputee and prosthetist can often become a very special one. Depending on the patient's age and health, many years of interaction with a prosthetist may follow the initial encounter. If, in the rare circumstance disagreements arise because of personality or demeanor, other services should be sought to assure the best possible immediate and long-term outcomes.

After surgery, patients should be fit with a shrinker or elastic bandage wrap. Much like a bodybuilder who stops lifting, normal muscle tissue deprived of a foot, knee, or hand to move will atrophy. This is a normal process, and occurs along with healing of the surgical site. The shrinker helps this process and aids in establishing future limb shape. The importance of this step cannot be overemphasized; failure to adequately shape and/or reduce a limb can result in more complicated and less successful fitting.

Depending on the patient and doctor, fitting can occur as soon as the day of surgery, or more commonly after four to six weeks. The initial visit will usually involve having some type of mold or measurement being taken to make a socket, the "cup" into which the residuum will fit. The second visit should be a fitting, where the socket fit and alignment (how the prosthesis is put together for optimal function) are determined. Depending on the particular situation, the patient will next receive the prosthesis in some form to begin gait training.

The type of prosthesis, along with the specific components chosen, will depend on various factors. Unfortunately, the reality of today's world is that insurance coverage may have some bearing on the prosthetic design. Insurers often make use of activity levels to determine what is appropriate for each insured. Individuals that are more active or those likely to reach higher levels tend to receive components that will allow for things such as running, jumping, varied cadence locomotion, and ascending/descending stairs. Prosthetic components, by their design, may improve an individual's ability to do certain things. However, some patients may not have coverage or need for many of the newest, high-tech items.

One of my core beliefs is that **a prosthesis does not walk by itself. An individual uses a prosthesis as a tool to reach his or her desired level of activity**. Any person who honestly works and strives to use a prosthesis will likely reach at least a minimum level of use. This result is independent of what components are used or even how the prosthesis is put together. Many a pirate is pictured with a peg leg (Fig. 1), and while we've come a long way since then, and a pirate may not have had the mobility desired by today's patient, independent function was achieved. Conversely, no matter what the fit or component selection, a patient unwilling to put forth the necessary effort will never reach his or her potential.

The pirate analogy is a good one for describing the prosthesis. Below the knee, a prosthesis is composed of three main parts: the socket, the pylon, and the foot as shown in Figures 2a and 2b. Most pirate peg legs lacked a foot, essential to provide improved leverage for balance and propulsion. Above the knee, an additional component is included—that of the knee (Fig. 2c).

Socket technology has changed over the years, but remains the same in many ways. The socket is designed to carry a patient's weight and to allow for the transmission of power and direction to the prosthesis. Most amputations are not designed to bear weight directly on the end of the limb. A Syme's amputation, or a disarticulation of the foot from the lower leg, is unique in this way. Amputees with this procedure may be able to walk without a prosthesis, directly on the healed

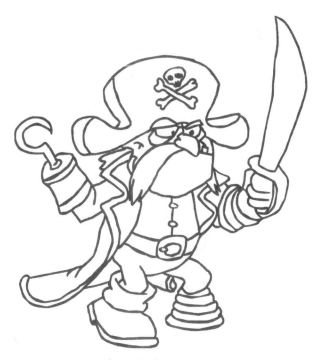

Figure 1 Pirate cartoon.

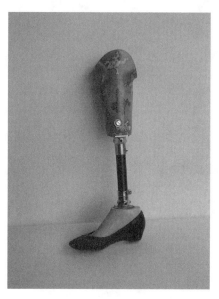

Figure 2a Example of a below-knee prosthesis socket, pylon, and foot.

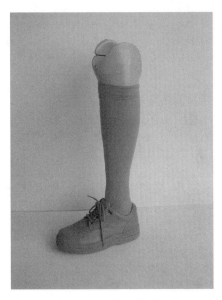

Figure 2b Example of a completed below-knee prosthesis.

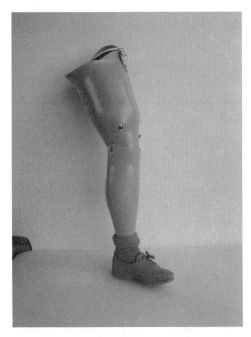

Figure 2c Example of a completed above-knee prosthesis socket, knee joint, calf, and foot.

extremity. This could be useful in emergencies or with restroom needs at night. However, my experience with this surgery is mixed, in that this function is only sometimes achieved. Many surgeries leave loose, unstable tissue that migrates in stance and causes pain. Others may have no cushion at all, only the boney distal tibia and fibula. The Syme's amputation may also present fewer options with component selection, as space is limited to only a few designs of feet.

Below the knee (transtibial), soft tissue areas are compressed and boney areas are relieved. Sockets are designed to spread body weight over the maximum allowable area, with less pressure applied to the often-problematic cut distal tibia and head of the fibula. The trim of the posterior socket should allow for relatively unrestricted range of motion while seated, up to approximately 100 degrees of flexion.

Above the knee (frequently referred to as transfemoral), the ischium, or "seat bone," becomes a weight-bearing point for most socket designs. Older quadrilateral socket designs have direct pressure to the ischium and are shaped with four distinct sides. Although not new, a quad socket may still be appropriate for more limited ambulators or wearers because they are much less technical in nature and may offer easier donning and use, especially if outside caretakers will be involved. More current designs, often called ischial containment or narrow M-L, have a more natural shape with some modifications to capture and hold the various muscles of the thigh. Compared to the quad socket, these are somewhat more intimate and precise in their fit. Most of these designs apply pressure along the lateral femur and contain the ischium inside the socket brim to maximize stability and control. Other than the cut end of the femur, the above-knee limb can be compressed almost entirely for maximum distribution of weight and pressure.

On some socket designs, an interface may be used to cushion and protect, or to allow for suspension (holding the prosthesis on). The older, standby interface is a sock. While providing a small level of cushion, the primary use of a sock is that of adjusting fit. Thicker or thinner socks are worn to compensate for daily weight and volume fluctuations. A liner may also be used, usually made with some variation of silicone or urethane. Liners can be made with different thicknesses (e.g., 3 mm, 6 mm), or can have the material be various thicknesses in different areas of the liner. The materials used reduce skin shear and offer a potential reduction in tissue stress by dispersing socket forces. They are rolled on, much like a condom, and may have an attachment point on the end for a pin. The pin is used to lock the liner and thus the patient into the prosthesis. This is regarded as a very secure method of prosthesis suspension (Figs. 3a and b). Without liners, suspension may be gained from suction or various straps, belts, or sleeves. Patient preference, skin integrity, manual dexterity, eyesight, comprehension, and residual

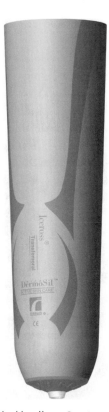

Figure 3a Suspension: locking liner. Courtesy of Ossur North America.

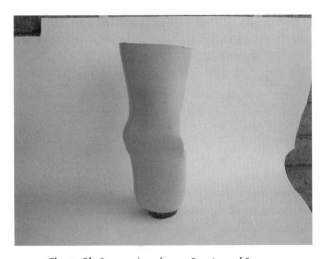

Figure 3b Suspension sleeve. Courtesy of Syncor.

limb shape/size should all be considered when the method of suspension or socket design is determined.

Prosthetic feet probably provide the widest variability in overall prosthetic function for below-knee patients. Very basic Solid Ankle Cushion Heel (SACH) feet (Fig. 4a) can be used for low-level walkers and vary little from 100-year-old designs. They are a block of wood covered with foot-shaped rubber. Energy-storing feet have some level of spring in them, and provide energy return to each step (Figs. 4b and c). They function much like a diving board, flexing and

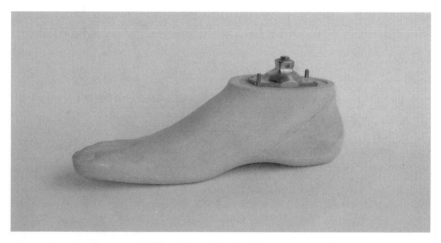

Figure 4a Industries SACH (solid ankle cushion heel) foot. Courtesy of Kingsley Manufacturing.

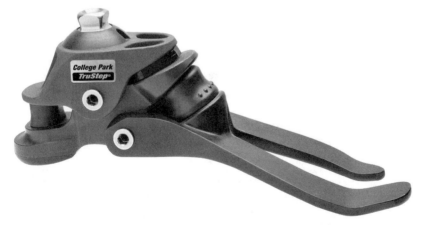

Figure 4b TruStep carbon foot multi-axis with bumper. Courtesy of College Park Industries.

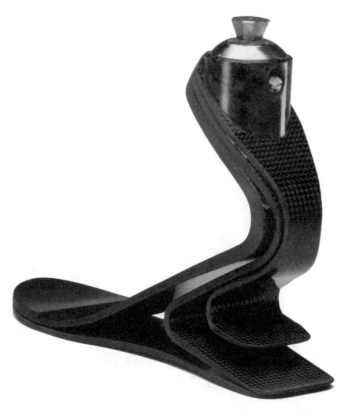

Figure 4c Renegade foot. (Courtesy of Freedom Innovations, Inc.)

returning during the weight-bearing portion of gait. They may have internal keels made of plastic or carbon fiber. Some feet also incorporate an ankle to allow for improved function on uneven terrain. This may seem intuitively necessary, but other considerations such as added weight may come into play. Increased complexity and mechanics may also necessitate more frequent maintenance.

The pylon, or the connection from the socket to the foot, is often a simple tube of aluminum or carbon. As an addition, some type of shock absorber may be added to reduce the impact of each step, functioning similarly to that on an automobile. This also adds to the overall weight, but many patients enjoy the mild bounce provided. Golfers or hikers may benefit from the addition of a rotational component that allows for torsion, or turning, of the foot relative to the socket. A spring, or resilient pylon absorbs shock and returns the foot to normal after the rotational forces are stopped. This can greatly reduce shear forces on the limb and may improve function in certain activities.

In an above-knee prosthesis, a knee unit is added. A knee not only allows for flexion in sitting, but also becomes an integral part of the design to provide stability during stance and to control the swing phase of gait. Many knees are available to choose from (Figs. 5a, b, and c), the most basic models function like a door hinge. Stability, or the ability of the prosthesis to resist buckling, is achieved by correct placement of the knee relative to the socket and foot. This is determined

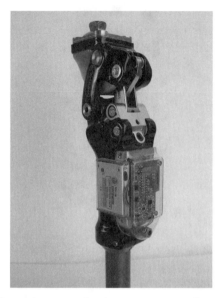

Figure 5a Polycentric Pneumatic Microprocessor Knee by DAW Industries.

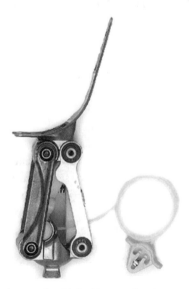

Figure 5b Four-bar knee unit with locking mechanism. Courtesy of Otto Bock.

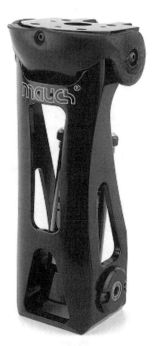

Figure 5c MAUCH hydraulic knee unit with frame. (Courtesy of Ossür North America.)

by the prosthetist during the fitting stage. A safety brake may be added to allow for binding of the joint in case of a stumble or misstep. Hydraulics in the form of oil or air may be included to better control the swing of the lower leg in varied cadences. They may also add to stability and allow for controlled flexing of the knee, as would be required in descending stairs step over step. The newest options include microprocessor control to instantly read and modify knee function in order to optimize swing, stability, and cadence. They may include batteries, which need charging regularly. They may also require scheduled maintenance, more so than lower technology devices.

As previously mentioned, the assembly of all these components is done in a scheduled fitting. It is at this time that changes are made to obtain optimum socket fit and alignment. Placement of the various components will profoundly change both the fit and function. A prosthesis in this state may not look good, but it is not supposed to. Devices to allow shift and angular changes may be incorporated, but will be taken out for finishing. If, and only if, positive results are achieved should the prosthesis progress to finishing. Otherwise, a second fitting may be needed to make changes. The end result of the fittings should be an agreement between the prosthetist and the amputee that everything feels good, with all goals of proper fit and alignment having been met.

It is difficult to quantify what the patient may feel, what good really is, or what is reasonable to expect. I have thought about this a great deal, and I feel confident in making the following statement: **The prosthesis should not hurt.** Many words can be used to describe what the new amputee may initially feel. Pressure, support, "newness," and tightness are all applicable. Pain or discomfort is not acceptable. Like all things new, time will smooth the new sensations and they will become more normal. The patient's body will adjust to the gradually increased duration of use and placement of body weight. Various methods can be used to improve socket comfort, including the use of check sockets (Figs. 6a and b), a clear device that allows for visual inspection by the prosthetist and is heat moldable for ease of adjustment at problem areas. This would be used in the fitting stage.

This is also the point at which patients should speak up if not satisfied with the results. Whether resolution of a concern can be made with a simple explanation or a change in componentry, this is the time. Easily made corrections or modifications at this time will become more difficult and costly later. The cosmetic considerations should also be reviewed at this time, as a variety of coverings are available, including "skins" made to look and feel natural as shown in Fig. 7.

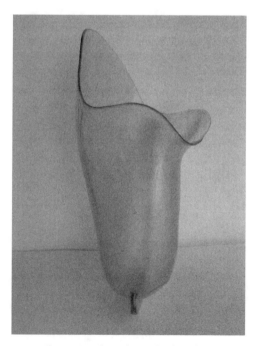

Figure 6a Above-knee check socket.

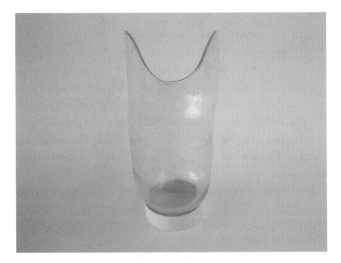

Figure 6b Below-knee check socket.

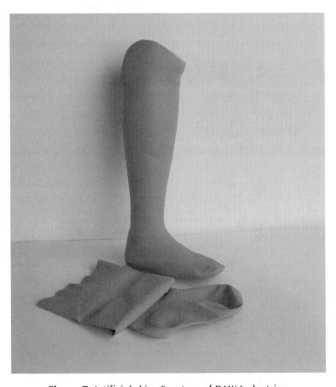

Figure 7 Artificial skin. Courtesy of DAW Industries.

Once the fitting is complete and final fabrication of the prosthesis has occurred, the amputee will begin functioning with the prosthesis. Some progress should be anticipated with the passing of each day, although it may take greater time intervals to better determine improvements gained. Visits to the prosthetist may be required for adjustments to the socket fit secondary to volume changes from atrophy or edema. It may also be necessary to adjust the alignment and function of the prosthesis as changes may occur in gait as the amputee begins to walk more. Patients may also be referred to physical therapy for strength, balance, and functional training. Both types of follow-up care are essential and can have profound effects on the outcome.

Skin integrity should be good with no abrasions or wounds. Problem areas may begin with areas of redness that linger more than 10 to 15 minutes after prosthesis removal. Diabetic neuropathy may affect sensation, so having patients not depend solely on sense of feel should be stressed. Eyesight may also be impaired, so while it is recommended to visually inspect the skin, others involved in care may need to assist. Check the used prosthetic socks, if worn next to the skin, for blood or fluid stains. Silicone liners may contain drainage or blood. Strong odors may indicate an unseen infection.

As time passes, strength, balance, and endurance should gradually improve. While there are no set time limits to reach goals or to plateau one's progress, each person should evaluate his or her own abilities and potential. This may include discussions with a doctor, therapist, or the prosthetist. An honest assessment of overall health is necessary to deduce probable outcomes. This should never be seen as a limiting factor, because many patients have far exceeded expectations. Although it may be difficult to discuss limitations, it should be acknowledged that not every amputee will reach a level of running and jumping. Television has added to many misconceptions regarding what can happen when someone is fit with a prosthesis. This may be interesting, and can certainly be held as a lofty goal for some. However, many others may not realistically reach these levels of activity.

Summary

A prosthesis should not be viewed as a death knell to independent lifestyles. Many patients, bedridden for years with open wounds or deformed limbs, have undergone amputation with a return to walking in 3 or 4 months. I have found the human desire to walk a very strong one. Ridding oneself of wheelchair dependence gives rise to the freedom of human locomotion, carrying items, improving self-image, and greater mobility with improved access to buildings and vehicles. With the aide of technology, personal motivation can result in marvelous accomplishments.

References

Bowker JH, Michael JW, Eds. *Atlas of Limb Prosthetics: Surgical, Prosthetic, and Rehabilitation Principles*, 2nd ed. St. Louis, MO: Mosby-Year Book, 2002.

Orthotics & Prosthetics Product Information, www.prosthetics-orthotics.com, 2006.

Smith DG, Michael JW, Bowker JH, Eds. *Atlas of Amputations and Limb Deficiencies: Surgical, Prosthetic, and Rehabilitation Principles*, 3rd ed. Rosemont IL: American Academy of Orthopaedic Surgeons, 2004.

Suggested Readings

O&P Digital Technologies. http://www.oandp.com, 2006.

Levy SW. *Skin Problems of the Amputee*. St. Louis, MO: Warren H. Green Publishers, 1982.

Sabolich J. *You're Not Alone*, revised edition, Oklahoma City, OK: Sabolich Prosthetic & Research Center, 1996.

10

Psychosocial and Psychophysiological Implications of Amputation

James Price, PhD, CPO, FAAOP

Disease and Amputation

Common medical knowledge implies that amputation due to disease is the ultimate result of insufficient vascular supply to the affected limb. The major contributor to vascular insufficiency resulting in limb amputation is diabetes (American Orthotic and Prosthetic Association 1999). This chapter focuses on the physiologically and psychologically complicating effects of diabetes as well as the implications of peripheral vascular disease as the two primary causes of limb amputation.

Vascular disruptions relating to the diabetic foot include neuropathic ulcers, gangrene, Charcot arthropathy, and microcirculatory disturbances resulting in uncontrollable edema. Each disruption commonly results in amputation of the affected limb because of the structural breakdown of body tissues and the inability for the tissues to regenerate due to compromised blood supply. Ulcers present as open wounds that cannot heal. Gangrene is necrotic tissue that proliferates if left unchecked. Charcot arthropathy is a collapse of the skeletal structure of the foot. Edema due to microvascular disease constricts circulation, which can eventually lead to any of the aforementioned disorders related to diabetes. In each of these cases, an absent pulse in the foot, followed by ischemia and ultimate tissue breakdown, precede invasive treatments.

Other risks associated with diabetes include peripheral vascular disease and coronary thrombosis. Coronary thrombosis is the leading cause of death in diabetics (Edmonds and Foster 1994). Those who suffer renal disease preceded by diabetes are predisposed to amputation after kidney transplant. Lifestyle-oriented risk factors for amputations in diabetics are smoking, obesity, insulin sensitivity, blood glucose control, and lipoprotein patterns (Grenfell 1994). Grenfell emphasizes hemostatic function as the culprit in diabetic disorders. Stagnancy in the bloodstream exacerbates the nature of the disease in that the accumulation of sugar in the blood and the attachment to proteins is the root problem.

Although diabetes is the major contributing malady of those who suffer limb loss, and is primarily responsible for vascular insufficiency leading to amputation, vascular disease does present apart from diabetes and ranks second as a cause for amputation by disease (American Orthotic and Prosthetic Association 1999). The underlying problem in vascular disease is venous stasis, a condition similar to the diabetic circulatory condition, yet being manifested void of the inefficient processing of insulin (McCarthy 1983). In venous stasis disorders there are stagnation of blood, bacterial growth, and ultimately infection. Lymphatic edema is a complicating condition of venous stasis and presents another similarity to the diabetic vascular condition. Predisposing factors to nondiabetic peripheral vascular disease are diet (high fat intake), lifestyle deficits (lack of physical exercise), and genetic influence such as the hereditary predisposition to a high percentage of low-density lipoproteins (bad cholesterol).

Educators should:

1. Advise the patient concerning the ubiquitous nature of diabetes and its effect on all body structures.
2. Promote awareness of the importance of positive lifestyle habits; including proper diet, sleep, and exercise.
3. Instruct the patient on proper skin care or refer the patient to someone who can provide guidance concerning skin care issues.

Psychological and Biopsychosocial Issues and the Phantom Phenomenon

Psychological issues of those suffering diabetic conditions are categorized by Jacobson and Leibovich (1985) as (a) psychosocial stress, (b) diabetic control, (c) environmental supports, and most importantly, (d) predictable phases of life crises. Jacobson and Leibovich present a model for understanding psychological issues faced by those with diabetes. The model includes the consideration of the risks that are present, personal abilities, and coping, and determines the individual's predisposition to being resilient or symptomatic. Individuals who follow the pattern of resiliency are able to better cope with the predictable phases of life crises that are associated with diabetes.

Gray (1983) examined social aspects of peripheral vascular disease. These categories can be added to psychosocial issues important to the diabetic and are pertinent constructs due to the influence of psychological conditions on pain perception. Aging and disease, education, religious attitudes, fearful attitudes, frustration, and resignation are considered instrumental in the resolution of social issues.

Once disease has progressed to the point that amputation becomes necessary, it is reasonable to expect that the victim of limb loss will have significant and complex issues to resolve. The pain associated with the disease has been replaced and sometimes coupled with the pain of surgery, and the psychological implications of disease have become psychological implications of body image and disease (Breakey 1997). One of these issues of immense complexity and profuse suffering is that of experiencing the phantom limb (Melzack and Wall 1988).

According to Melzack and Wall (1988), phantom limb pain is the most terrible and fascinating of all clinical pain syndromes. Melzack and Wall claim that the experience of the phantom limb is not always described as painful, yet the sensation of the missing limb being intact after amputation is extremely prevalent. Phantom limb sensation has been shown to be present in 65% of amputees six months after amputation, and in 60% at two-year and seven-year intervals (Melzack and Wall 1988). Pinel (2000) reports that 50% of amputees experience phantom pain classified as chronic or severe. In the Melzack and Wall research, the phantom limb experience was characterized as one of pain or void of pain and categorized as phantom limb sensation.

The majority of amputees report phantom limb sensation immediately after surgery. It is described as a tingling feeling in which the original shape of the extremity is perceived. The phantom limb reacts the same when moving, sitting, and lying down, and the tendency for the missing extremity to feel present has caused some amputees to step out of bed expecting their foot to touch the floor, or to reach out to grasp an object with a missing hand. With time, the shape of the phantom extremity begins to change and Melzack and Wall describe a "telescoping" effect in which the foot or hand begins to recede back into the body until it seems to be attached right at the stump. In some cases, the phantom foot or hand subsequently disappears. Melzack and Wall suggest that the central nervous system produces the phantom in response to lack of normal input and that it manifests as a neural substrate of our perception of body position.

Phantom pain is described as cramping, shooting, burning, or crushing and is reported on a broad spectrum from occasionally to frequently in those who experience it. The pain may vary with respect to quality and intensity. Rather than simply feeling the shape of the absent extremity, those who suffer phantom limb pain report the feeling that the appendage is contorted. Phantom pain can be triggered by emotional upsets as well as bodily functions.

The research of Melzack and Wall (1988) concerning phantom pain has been extensive. They have determined that phantom pain may endure long after the tissue damaged from disease and surgery has healed and that "trigger zones" may spread to healthy areas of the body.

Melzack (1989) maintains that the experience of the phantom limb is realistic to the limb loss patient because the same brain processes that are present when the body is intact remain present after amputation. Melzack describes the body as being unitary with an integrated quality that includes the self and the incorporation of a neural network that can be changed by sensory experience although the "body-self" is genetically determined. Melzack describes experiences of the body as having a quality of self, thereby influencing the individual's perception and response to pain.

There is ample controversy in determining the causal mechanisms of phantom limb sensation. The major problem is the attempt to identify a single problem as the entire explanation when it is more likely that there are a variety of contributing factors. Melzack and Wall (1988) suggest that theories emphasizing a progression from the periphery to the central nervous system as a means of explaining the phantom limb phenomenon are inadequate. According to Melzack and Wall, more than 40 types of therapy to address phantom limb pain have been developed, with a meager success rate of 15%. This is understandably frustrating to the individual who suffers limb loss. It is more frustrating to the individual who has experienced disease and pain resulting in amputation only to experience little or no relief once the amputation is performed. This low success rate is indicative of a predominant ignorance of the mechanisms that underlie phantom limb pain.

Melzack (1989) cites psychological evidence that perceptual experience is influenced by past history and current state of mind. In other words, state of mind, or emotion, under certain circumstances may determine responses to pain or pain sensation thresholds. Melzack adds that phantom limb pain perplexes the investigation by beginning as signals of serious body damage and may persist, spread, and increase in intensity to the point that it becomes a malady in its own right because the pain may become worse than the original injury that caused it. He goes on to say that phantom limb pain is more likely in those who have suffered pain prior to amputation. Evidence reveals that prolonged pain can have deleterious effects resulting in immunosuppression due to extended periods of stress, anxiety, or depression (Kludt 2000).

Educators should:

1. Discuss phantom limb or phenomena issues with amputee patients.
2. Investigate alternatives for management of phantom pain for the patient.
3. Explore emotional and social variables with the patient that might contribute to phantom pain and distress.

Pain, Stress, and Immunologic Compromise

Critical to the diabetic patient are the effects of pain and stress on the immune system. Immune dysfunction has been examined by Vedhara, Fox, and Wang (1999), who concluded that the consequences of stress on the immune system can be profound. Vedhara et al. investigated immunologic response by exploring lymphocyte subsets and proliferation, cytokine levels, and cytotoxicity assays, virus and viral components including antigen detection. According to Kemeny and Laudenslager (1999), there are measurable differences in the immune systems in both humans and animals under conditions of stress. The authors provide a reminder that individual patterns of affective, behavioral, and cognitive responses significantly influence reaction to stress and physiologic consequences. Whether the stress is classified as a major or minor event also may play an important role in the immune response.

The work of Tracey, Walker, and Carmody (2000) provides evidence that the stress-pain connection may be a reciprocal event. Not only does pain produce stress, which contributes to immunologic consequences, but also prolonged stress may produce a predisposition to chronic pain. This is supported by Bragdon (2000), who studied the stress responses of individuals suffering from temporomandibular pain, and by Moxham (1999), who investigated pain in fibromyalgia patients experiencing the stress of unrestorative sleep. Interestingly, the Bragdon study revealed a correlation between depression and pain sensitivity with blunted cortisol stress response. Cortisol excretion promotes basic survival functions including quick thinking, fast reflexes, and increased strength. All are components of the fight or flight response. It is important to recognize that while excessive amounts of cortisol can actually produce stress, small amounts of the hormone are necessary to ensure proper glucose metabolism, insulin release for blood sugar maintenance, and proper immune function. The Moxham study revealed a cyclic event in which unrestorative sleep contributed to fatigue, which mediated pain. Another fibromyalgia study presented stress as a predictor of both pain and depression (Kim 2000). Similarly, life stress and depression have been associated with experiences of chronic pain (Catley 2000). Specific to the phantom phenomenon, Angrilli and Koester (2000) provide evidence as to the impact of stress on pain intensity and suggest a connection between the long-term emotional memory of amputation and the occurrence of phantom pain. In the Angrilli and Koester study, cardiovascular hyperactivity was observed during the reports of subjects concerning their amputation experience.

Other examples of stress producing pain with physiological consequences include work-related stress and musculoskeletal pain with catecholamine compromises, elevated blood pressure, increased heart rate, and psychosomatic symptoms (Lundberg et al. 1999); chronic psychoemotional stress and reduced pain thresholds (Ashkinazi and Vershinina 1999); stress producing injury and resulting in prolonged chronic pain (Melzack 1998); posttraumatic stress disorder, alterations of hypothalamic adrenal axis, and chronic pain (Heim et al. 1998); and the development of pain in pain-free subjects after prolonged mental stress (Bansevicius, Westgaard, and Jensen 1997). Specifically pertinent to the diabetic patient is evidence suggesting that degenerative disease processes combined with major stress-producing constructs such as bereavement have been shown to result in immunologic decrement (Burkhalter 1998).

Educators should:

1. Provide information to the patient about immunosuppression and the complicating effects of diabetes.
2. Discuss stress-reduction techniques and/or provide resources for stress management for the patient.
3. Discuss with the patient the potential implications of stress regarding pain and phantom pain and vice versa.

Depression and Disability

Depression is defined as "a state of low mental vitality" or "dejection" (*New Lexicon Webster's Dictionary of the English Language* 1992). Hay, Hay, and Sperry (1998) describe depression as a generic term that has been used to explain a variety of disorders. Situational and biological depression may present interactively or exclusively in related or unrelated phenomena. Depression in the elderly is generally reported differently than the depression of middle-aged or younger counterparts specifically with increased somatic concerns and less guilt. Hypochondriasis, psychotic depression, and pseudodementia are more prevalent with age. Physical illnesses, sociological considerations, and other psychological concerns may also play an interactive role.

The following themes are consistent in many individuals diagnosed as depressed:

1. Depressed mood most of the day nearly every day.
2. Markedly diminished interest or pleasure in all or almost all activities most of the day.
3. Significant weight loss or weight gain.
4. Insomnia or hypersomnia nearly every day.
5. Psychomotor agitation or retardation nearly every day.
6. Fatigue or loss of energy nearly every day.
7. Feelings of worthlessness or excessive or inappropriate guilt.
8. Diminished ability to think or concentrate.
9. Recurrent thoughts of death, suicidal ideation, or a suicide attempt.

The aforementioned characteristics have remained static over time for determining depression and were utilized as a basis for diagnosis in the *Diagnostic and Statistical Manual of Mental Disorders*, 3rd ed. [DSM-III]. The newer version, DSM-IV-TR, no longer states a requirement of the presence of five of these characteristics; however, the same qualities remain inherent in determining higher and lower levels of depression as well as depressive symptoms as defined by the more recent manual. According to Albus, Dozier, and Stovall (1999), major depression might be genetically determined.

Individuals who are diagnosed as depressed may exhibit depression in any or all stages of the life cycle (Greenspan and Pollock 1998). Furthermore, depression may be manifested prior to, during, or just after major life events. Onset of disability is a salient example of major life events that produce depression. Whitbourne's (1998) characterization of physical identity in which appearance, competence, and limitations combine to develop a sense of self depends heavily on the individual's capability to function physically. Physical impairment may arise from trauma or from the results of disease.

The predisposition of the elderly to physical disease justifies investigating to what extent compromise of well-being is mediated by disease. Dent et al. (1999) suspected that the incidence of disease revealed few independent connections with depressive symptoms in older people, whereas disability produced a marked impact on depressive symptoms in every circumstance. In other words, physical disease may not always lead to disability; however, when it does it is usually followed by depressive symptoms. Ormel et al. (1997) support this finding by asserting that the nature of the physical condition does not determine psychological distress; however, the severity of the disability along with availability of psychological resources and personality traits of the affected individual does. In a study concerning correlates of depression in older adults, Roberts et al. (1997) found that healthy elderly individuals are at no greater risk of depression than younger adults; however, older adults with physical health problems or disability are.

Landreville and Gervais (1997) state that depression is the most frequent type of psychological distress that occurs subsequent to disability. Elderly people who are depressed have a significant amount of co-morbidity such as physical disability (Katona, Manela, and Livingston 1997). Katona, Manela, and Livingston maintain that the majority of elderly people with depression receive no pharmacological treatment and surmise that primary physical or psychiatric symptoms may obscure the diagnosis of depression.

A study by Langer (1994) revealed that among the various types of disabilities exhibited by her subjects, amputees displayed more indecisiveness, thoughts of death, and thoughts of self-harm. Rybarczk, Szymanski, and Nicholas (2000) discuss the need for amputees to come to terms with loss of limb as well as consequential functional limitations.

Restriction of activity is interrelated with public self-consciousness and depression (Williamson 1995; Williamson et al. 1994). Williamson (1995) determined that amputees who exhibited restricted levels of activities were reluctant to go out in public because of feelings of self-consciousness, and at the same time felt vulnerable and less able to defend themselves. Perceived social stigma has been found to contribute significantly to depression (Rybarczyk et al. 1995). Rybarczyk et al. (2000) outline a broad spectrum of psychological responses of the amputee that range from extreme despair to feelings of relief after eliminating the source of pain.

Perceptual changes after amputation are a potential source of emotional despair (Knecht et al. 1996). Knecht et al. determined by magnetic source imaging that organizational and perceptual changes correlated with the number of sites from which painful stimuli could evoke referred sensation. The work of Knecht et al. gives insight into the psychophysiological influences of amputation by revealing that phantom sensations can be evoked by stimulating sites adjacent to the amputation site as well as stimulating certain points on the face. This relates to the work of Melzack and Wall (1988), who reported that phantom limb pain can mediate depressive symptoms, especially when the phantom limb is evoked by unrelated body functions.

Modification of the sense of self, sense of loss, awareness of mortality, loss of confidence, disfigurement, loss of balance, guilt, and phantom limb sensations are among the traumatic effects of amputation that can cause this population to have a bleak outlook for the future (McGarry 1993). McGarry places a sense of urgency on the importance of the development of coping strategies to promote positive social change through addressing the issues of the limb loss population.

Educators should:

1. Discuss the potential for distress to develop as a result of the disease process.
2. Identify various contributors to the development of depressive symptoms.
3. Advise patients about available resources for management of stressful situations.
4. Discuss the importance of identifying proper expectations related to the disease process.

Health Promotion and Social Change

Dunn (2000) maintains that social psychological aspects are undeniably linked to issues concerning rehabilitation because coping, adaptation, and responses to these issues are determined by the social perception, judgment, and action of the perceiver. Perhaps the most salient point of Dunn's position is with respect to perception, and according to Dunn, the experience of disability as perceived by the affected individual may be influenced by personality characteristics.

Personality characteristics can have significant influences on the ability to adapt to (cope with) specific circumstances. Coping strategy has been shown to mediate adjustment to prosthesis use in amputees (Gallagher and MacLachlan 1999). Friedman, Hawley, and Tucker (1994) provide an overview of the dichotomous categorization of adapting personalities. Specifically, the "disease-prone" personality is characterized by (a) perfectionism, (b) introversion, (c) procrastination, (d) external locus of control, (e) nonbelief in a just world, (d) low self-efficacy, (e) pessimism, (f) negativity, (g) outcomes avoidance, (h) neuroticism, (i) maladjusted personality, (j) low self-esteem, (k) unsure tendencies, and (l) dependency. The "self-healing" personality is characterized by a preponderance of the opposite of the aforementioned qualities of the disease-prone personality and, according to Baron and Byrne (2000), has a less difficult time developing coping abilities. Furthermore, Baron and Byrne assert that most people fall somewhere along a continuum between the two personality types, with those positioned closer to the disease-prone personality on the continuum having the most difficulty.

For those who have personality types that gravitate away from the self-healing category, attention should be given to strategies that promote positive methods of dealing with stress, as well as general coping with negative circumstances. Baron and Byrne (2000) provide an overview of the application of social psychological strategies to health-related behaviors. The authors stress the importance of consistent positive lifestyle habits that include nutritious foods, adequate sleep, and regular exercise.

Those faced with overcoming the detrimental psychological effects of a disabling condition frequently find themselves in the pivotal position of requiring lifestyle change. Various studies suggest that exercise, and specifically intensity of exercise, is a predictor of self-efficacy, while self-efficacy has been shown to predict positive lifestyle behaviors such as exercise.

According to Winett (1998), the most effective exercise programs are those that include high-intensity activities. Winett calls attention to the recent promotion by psychologists of high-volume activity programs and notes that the time-consuming nature of such programs results in the predictable outcome of nonmaintenance. Winett stresses that the high-intensity exercise theory leads to greater potential for "self-mastery" and "self-efficacy." Self-mastery being the control an individual acquires through positive lifestyle practices, while self-efficacy is the state of well-being that results after developing that control. Jessor, Turbin, and Costa (1998) support the notion that 15 minutes of exercise per day, or even every other day, is enough to increase fitness, well-being, and self-efficacy.

Acute bouts of exercise produce self-efficacy changes and consequential feelings of well-being, and reduce perceptions of fatigue and psychological distress (Mihalko, McAuley, and Bane 1996). The significance of understanding the efficacy change process is demonstrated by Mullan and Markland (1997), who studied individuals participating in exercise programs. Self-determination was identified as a prominent characteristic of behavioral regulation, and the authors endorse motivational considerations relating to the process of change.

Self-efficacy contributes significantly to predicting exercise behavior. Those who have high levels of self-efficacy may adapt to disability more proficiently by virtue of emotion-based coping. Proper training and education after the onset of disability might help boost self-efficacy and consequential success concerning rehabilitation intervention through problem-based coping.

Recent research provides insight into the importance of positive health behaviors such as exercise, diet, and proper sleep; however, these behaviors are generally considered strategies that help to circumvent the negative effects of stress. To complete a thorough investigation of social psychological tactics for positive behavior, specific coping strategies of a social psychological nature should be examined. For instance, Compas et al. (1991) outlined a two-level process of coping, coping being defined as an effective response to stress. Emotion-focused coping is compared to problem-focused coping with the former being an attempt to deal with negative feelings and the latter involving a focus on threat and gaining control of that threat. According to Baron and Byrne (2000), those who tend to cope through the problem-focused method are generally those who are identified as having self-healing personalities. Baron and Byrne discuss regulatory control, which is a coping tactic that involves thought control, control over feelings, control over actions, and direction of energy and attention. Creating positive affect is discussed as a method of counteracting negative emotions that are the potential producers of stress, anxiety, and subsequent depression.

Gallagher and MacLachlan (2000) determined that those who found positive meaning in the experience of amputation demonstrated more favorable adjustment to limitations, physical capabilities, health ratings, and athletic aptitude. Examples might include individuals who have entered "helping" professions because of exposure to those professions as a result of their own disease experience, those who have become involved in amputee athletics as a result of amputation, or those who have conquered specific lifestyle deficits (drug abuse, sedentary lifestyles, emotionally destructive behavior, etc.) after becoming disabled.

The capacity for an individual to exhibit resilience may be determined by various influences such as education, income, and occupational status; however, according to Ryff et al. (1998), the reflection of resilience is evident in the ultimate outcome of mind-body integration regardless of sociodemographic variables. Mind-body integration in this respect involves concern with positive mental strategies such as not becoming depressed, anxious, or physically ill in the face of adversity, as well as positive physical strategies such as diet, exercise, sleep, and aerobic capacities. Positive self-appraisal in spite of objective decline is cited as an important dynamic for maintenance of the sense of well-being (Borchelt et al. 1999). Participation in religious activities is purported by Koenig (1994) to result in "successful aging" regardless of physical health or environmental conditions.

Friendships and social networks have been shown to be essential aspects of an individual's support system (Cavenaugh 1998). Support systems, while important to all disabled, become even more valuable to the disabled elderly. Gallagher, Allen, and MacLachlan (2001) found that absence of support prior to amputation correlated with phantom limb pain after amputation. In a similar qualitative study, Gallagher and MacLachlan (2001) used a focus group methodology to examine adjustment to amputation. Support among others was found to be important in the adjustment process. It has been determined that the single most positive experience for a new amputee is communication and interaction with other amputees (Foort 1974).

The perception of minimal support has been shown to correlate with depressive symptoms and reduced quality of life in elderly individuals with physical impairments (Newsom and Schultz 1996). Each member of a social network has a distinct character, yet there is a simultaneous context that influences and is influenced by the individual, consequently setting the parameters of group social change (Stones 1992). Members of social networks who are initially strangers begin to relate to each other because of their commonalities (Brown 1995). Longino and Mittelmark (1996) emphasize the importance of sociodemographic dimensions as well as social resources as mechanisms that link the social environment to health status. This implies that the support of friends, siblings, and others can have a positive effect on physical health by reducing the potential for stress and anxiety brought on by isolation, and is supported by the work of Antonucci and Akiyama (1997) who state that social relations are associated with reduced morbidity. Similarly, Antonucci and Akiyama cite longitudinal studies in which people reporting the existence of high-quality social relationships had reduced rates of mortality between times of follow-up compared to those who did not.

Just as social support is associated with physical health, Antonucci and Akiyama maintain that there is empirical evidence supporting an association between positive social relations and mental competence in old age. The most significant supporters identified by the elderly were the spouse (if alive), children, siblings, and friends. Antonucci and Akiyama determined that the most valuable types of support given were (a) confiding, (b) reassurance, (c) respect, (d) sick care, and (e) conversation concerning problems and health.

Comprehensive amputee programs can provide the opportunity for amputees to participate in a network that provides peer counseling to new amputees. This type of network potentially provides a much-needed service for new patients, and gives participants a sense of purpose, a primary component for addressing their own needs. Involvement enables individuals to avoid feelings of being disenfranchised by reconceptualizing their lives and maintaining a sense of place and continuity of identity. Patients who have remained uninvolved tend to exhibit more distress and less communicative effort.
Educators should:

1. Examine with the patient the roles of personality and perception in response to disability.
2. Discuss the relationship between positive lifestyle practices and self-efficacy.
3. Help the patient to understand the concept of "positive meaning in disease experience" as well as ways to apply positive meaning in social network strategies.

Education and Patient-Practitioner Communication

Illness and medical treatment can be stressful from various standpoints. The patient has been thrust into the unknown, so to speak, and has to deal not only with the illness from a prognostic view, or the pain of the illness, but the contemplation of treatment for the illness and the thoughts that are generated from such contemplation. Wills and DePaulo (1991) assert that the decision to seek medical help is a coping mechanism in and of itself. In fact, it may be the first step in taking control of the situation through a problem-focused strategy, and the first step in self-education from which control may be manifested.

Rall, Peskoff, and Byrne (1994) support the concept of individuals learning as much as possible about their particular conditions to enhance sense of control, and consequently well-being. Learning as much as possible about the condition by seeking out those with similar problems is imperative.

> Patients should make it their hobby to educate themselves in the newest areas of medicine that affect their particular condition. They should read, write, and seek professionals who can make a difference in their lives by helping them be successful (Ratto 1991, p. 88).

Rall et al. conducted a study of 444 adults concerning perceptions of physicians and patient interaction and determined that the perception of the physician's information-giving behavior elicited positive affective and evaluative ratings. This showcases the need for positive communication between clinicians and patients.

Thompson, Nanni, and Levine (1994) identify perceived control as instrumental in coping with illness and other potentially stressful situations. Thompson, Nanni, and Levine investigated various levels of control with their subjects and identified two dimensions of control; primary versus secondary and central versus consequence-related control. All levels of perceived control were correlated with better adjustment and low depression. These findings are supported by Griffin and Rabkin (1998), who examined perceptions of control over illness and psychological adjustment. In the study, perceptions of control were associated with fewer depressive symptoms and less anxiety regarding death. The results of these studies are consistent with the results of Lachman and Weaver (1998), who investigated perception of control across various socioeconomic classes. The study revealed through multiple-regression analyses that higher perceived mastery and lower perceived constraints correlated with better health, life satisfaction, and lower depressive symptoms regardless of income group.

It has been suggested that another moderating coping influence is the availability of choice (Paterson and Neufeld 1995). Paterson and Neufeld evaluated 278 subjects by providing the availability of various courses of action in some scenarios versus the elimination of choice in others. It was determined that situations are viewed as more stressful when it is necessary to select coping options blindly or when significant information must be processed within a short period of time to determine a prospective coping option. This finding becomes more significant when the variable of disability is introduced. Specifically, those faced with the prospect of amputation may initially feel that the ability to choose has been eliminated. Applying the principles of Paterson and Neufeld, the perception of choice after amputation surgery then becomes crucial to psychological recovery. Dunn (1996) determined that amputees who found positive meaning in disabling experiences achieved higher levels of well-being.

While many aspects of the physical, emotional, and social domains that impact coping during and after the initial rehabilitation process are to a certain degree under the patient's control, examination of a holistic continuum representing a collaborative and comprehensive approach to patient management would not be complete without investigating those issues for which the patient has little or no control. Within the social domain there are many subcategories instrumental in contributing to the continuity and quality of the patient's care and involve clinician-patient interaction via nonverbal communication and various learning methods.

The purpose of this discussion is to examine techniques that can be employed and interpreted by the practitioner and that provide potentially positive influences on the practitioner-patient relationship. Symbolism and multiple intelligences theory are presented as gateways to positive rapport and potential patient adjustment. While beneficial to virtually all patient populations, these techniques might be particularly helpful in the management of the disabled, including those who suffer limb loss or other physical or emotional trauma.

A symbol is "any entity that can denote or refer to another entity" (Gardner 1993, p. 301). Gardner speaks of how various images, elements, or words are used to stand for "real-life" objects in the world and asserts that language alone cannot satisfy requirements for conveying thoughts. Without being aware, individuals tend to express feelings without using words (Lopicic-Pericic 1996). Facial expressions, gestures, look, voice, silence, posture, and movement are virtually continuous replacements for conventional linguistics.

In examining body knowledge as well as body prejudice as they relate to practitioner–patient interaction, cultural variables, biological considerations, and environment all seem to play an important part in how nonverbal communication takes place. According to Edelstein and Schein (1997), body image becomes a significant part of this equation for those who suffer limb loss. Edelstein and Schein maintain that self-esteem, anxiety, and life satisfaction are correlated with perception of body image, and it is understandable that a compromise in this perception interferes with nonverbal communication that depends on body knowledge. This is supported by Cleveland and Fisher (1978), who found that amputees as well as stroke victims have altered body images, necessitating the careful interpretation of signals. Stroke victims sometimes are restricted to using nonverbal communication, and even when the right hemisphere of the brain has been affected (which generally results in intact speech but impaired motor function), it is imperative that nonverbal cues are interpreted with care. Using symbolism in professional practice and practicing a variety of communication skills in patient management can be further explored through an evaluation of the theory of multiple intelligences.

The theory of multiple intelligences posits that intelligence is more than a single property of the mind and that multiplicity may be evident within creativity, leadership, and morals (Gardner 1999). Just as social structures within cultures exhibit a variety of nonverbal communicative skills, individuals within those cultures are purveyors of their own unique way of communicating thoughts and utilize methods that reflect major focuses or interests in their lives to convey those thoughts. One example of this type of unique communication style might be a patient who happens to be a pilot and uses a lower-limb prosthesis. In an attempt to describe how the prosthesis is responding during gait, the patient describes a "three-stage landing," a term familiar to pilots. The pilot is relating the "landing" of the prosthesis to the landing of an airplane. Torff and Gardner (1999) describe a vertical theory of intelligence in which separate cognitive mechanisms are utilized to address particular kinds of information or tasks. This is in contrast to horizontal theories of intelligence, which emphasize the mind's handling of tasks through a single, centralized system. The pilot who describes the response of the prosthesis as a three-stage landing might use other personal experience to describe additional aspects of the prosthesis. For instance, if the prosthesis squeaks, the patient might use language that reflects knowledge of music. For instance, "My prosthesis hits a high C whenever my heel contacts the floor." The communication techniques of each individual are a product of how learning has taken place during the life cycle.

Snyder (2000) found that 81% of participants in a study on learning styles were tactile/kinesthetic learners who prefer actually doing things as opposed to listening and watching during efforts to learn. This suggests that learners in any population should be assessed to determine the most effective manner of teaching them. Identification of multiple intelligences can be a basis for discovering strengths, minimizing weaknesses, and lead to realistic goal interventions. Educators should:

1. Advise patients as to the importance of communication between patients and practitioners as well as the importance of willingness to communicate.
2. Discuss the various methods of human communication including verbal and nonverbal cues.
3. Review the significance of "choice" and "control" of the patient in coping with disease and disability.

Summary

The topics presented in this chapter, while covering a broad spectrum, exemplify the essence of an approach that includes physical, social, and emotional constructs in addressing the needs of those who experience disease and limb loss.

Disease and amputation, immunologic compromise, and health-promotion strategies have an overarching physical theme; however, social and emotional implications can be found within these categories. A salient example is biopsychosocial concerns, which involve the physical, social, and emotional realms. Yet another example of the meshing of domains is the phantom phenomenon, which has physical and emotional origins and social ramifications. Likewise, mental resilience, personal control, self-efficacy, and stress and anxiety are emotional or psychological constructs that are affected by physical and social influence. Finally, education, support systems, body image, and clinician–client interaction are social-centered, but are influenced by physical and emotional stimuli.

The continua represented by each psychophysiological category of inquiry (physical, social, and emotional), and the tendency of each domain to cross the boundaries of other domains, highlights the holistic perspective and supports the philosophies of multidimensional support and multidimensional care in clinical patient management.

References

Albus, KE, Dozier, M, Stovall, KC. Attachment and psychopathology in adulthood. In J Cassidy, PR Shaver, Eds., *Handbook of Attachment: Theory, Research, and Clinical Applications.* New York: The Guilford Press, 1999, p. 497–519.

American Orthotic and Prosthetic Association. *Cost Factors in Prosthetics and Orthotics* [Brochure]. Alexandria, VA: American Orthotic and Prosthetic Association, 1999.

Angrilli, A, Koester, U. Psychophysiological stress responses in amputees with and without phantom limb pain. *Physiol Behav* 68(5):699–706, 2000.

Antonucci, TC, Akiyama, H. Social support and the maintenance of competence. In SL Willis, KW Schaie, M Hayward, Eds., *Societal Mechanisms for Maintaining Competence in Old Age.* New York: Springer Publishing Company, 1997, p. 182–206.

Ashkinazi, IY, Vershinia, EA. Pain sensitivity in chronic psychoemotional stress in humans. *Neurosci Behav Physiol* 29(3):333–337, 1999.

Bansevicius, D, Westgaard, RH, Jensen, C. Mental stress of long duration: EMG activity, perceived tension, fatigue, and pain development in pain-free subjects. *Headache* 37(8):499–510, 1997.

Baron, RA, Byrne, D. *Social Psychology* (9th ed.). Boston: Allyn and Bacon, 2000.

Borchelt, M, Gilberg, R, Horgas, AL, Geiselmann, B. On the significance of morbidity and disability in old age. In PB Baltes, KU Mayer, Eds., *The Berlin Aging Study: Aging from 70 to 100.* New York: Cambridge University Press, 1999, p. 403–429.

Bragdon, EE. Cardiovascular and pain responses to stress in healthy adults and temporo-mandibular disorder patients. (Doctoral dissertation, University of North Carolina, Chapel Hill). *Diss Abstr Int* 60(12-B):6410, 2000.

Breakey, JW. Body image: The lower limb amputee. *J Prosthet Orthot* 9(2):58–66, 1997.

Brown, DW. *When Strangers Cooperate: Using Social Conventions to Govern Ourselves.* New York: The Free Press, 1995.

Burkhalter, JE. A bereavement support group intervention: Effects on bereavement-specific situational coping and associations of dispositional coping style and situational coping with psychological distress and immune function in bereaved HIV seronegative gay men. (Doctoral dissertation, University of Miami). *Diss Abstr Int* 59(2-B):0865, 1998.

Catley, D. Psychological distress in chronic pain: Examination of integrative models of stress, and a cognitive-behavioral mediation model of depression. (Doctoral dissertation, New York University, Stony Brook). *Diss Abstr Int* 60(8-B):4207, 2000.

Cavenaugh, JC. Friendships and social networks among older people. In IH Nordhus, GR VandenBos, S Berg, P Fromholt, Eds., *Clinical Geropsychology.* Washington, DC: American Psychological Association, 1998, p. 137–140.

Cleveland, SE, Fisher, S. The role of body image in the psychoneuroses and psychoses. In SE Cleveland, S Fisher, Eds., *Body Image Pers.* Princeton, NJ: Van Nostrand 1958, p. 230–249.

Compas, BE, Banez, GA, Malcarne, V, Worsham, N. Perceived control and coping with stress: A developmental perspective. *J Soc Issues* 47(4):23–34, 1991.

Dent, OF, Waite, LM, Bennett, HP, Casey, BJ, Grayson, DA, Cullen, JS, Creasey, H, Broe, GA. A longitudinal study of chronic and depressive symptoms in a community sample of older people. *Aging Men Health* 3(4):351–357, 1999.

Dunn, DS. Well-being following amputation: Salutary effects of positive meaning, optimism, and control. *Rehabil Psychol* 41(4):285–302, 1996.

Dunn, DS. Social psychological issues in disability. In RG Frank, TT Elliott, Eds., *Handbook of Rehabilitation.* Washington, DC: American Psychological Association, 2000, p. 565–584.

Edelstein, J, Schein, JD. 1997 Body image: The lower-limb amputee. *J Prosthet Orthot* 9:58–66, 1997.

Edmonds, ME, Foster, AVM. The diabetic foot. In JC Pickup, G Williams, Eds., *Chronic Complications of Diabetes.* London: Blackwell Scientific Publications, 1994, p. 231–239.

Foort, J. How amputees feel about amputation. *Orthot Prosthet* 28:21–27, 1974.

Friedman, HS, Hawley, PH, Tucker, JS. Personality, health, and longevity. *Curr Dir Psychol Sci* 3(2):37–41, 1994.

Gallagher, P, Allen, D, MacLachlan, M. Phantom limb pain and residual limb pain following lower limb amputation: A descriptive analysis. *Disabil Rehabil* 23(12):522–530, 2001.

Gallagher, P, MacLachlan, M. Psychological adjustment and coping in adults with prosthetic limbs. *Behav Med* 25(3):117–124, 1999.

Gallagher, P, MacLachlan, M. Positive meaning in amputation and thoughts about the amputated limb. *Prosthet Orthot Int* 24:196–204, 2000.

Gallagher, P, MacLachlan, M. Adjustment to an artificial limb: A qualitative perspective. *J Health Psychol* 6(1):85–100, 2001.

Gardner, H. *Frames of Mind: The Theory of Multiple Intelligences.* New York: Basic Books, 440.

Gardner, H. *Intelligence Reframed: Multiple Intelligences for the 21st century.* New York: Basic Books, 292.

Gray, JAM. Social aspects of peripheral vascular disease. In ST McCarthy, Eds., *Peripheral Vascular Disease in the Elderly.* New York: Churchill Livingstone, 1983, pp. 191–199.

Greenspan, SI, Pollock, GH. *The Course of Life, Vol. VII.* Madison, CT: International Universities Press, 1998.

Grenfell, A. Clinical features and management of established diabetic nephropathy. In JC Pickup, G Williams (Eds.), *Chronic Complications of Diabetes.* Boston: Blackwell Scientific Publications, 1994, p. 169–191.

Griffin, KW, Rabkin, JG. Perceived control over illness, realistic acceptance, and psychological adjustment in people with AIDS. *J Soc Clin Psychol* 17(4):407–424, 1998.

Hay, DP, Hay, L, Sperry, L. Depression and anxiety in the elderly. In SI Greenspan, GH Pollock, Eds., *The Course of Life, Vol. VII.* Madison, CT: International Universities Press, Inc., 1998.

Heim, C, Ehlert, U, Hanker, JP, Hellhammer, DH. Abuse-related posttraumatic stress disorder and alterations of the hypothalamic-pituitary-adrenal axis in women with chronic pelvic pain. *Psychosom Med* 60(3):309–318, 1998.

Jacobson, AM, Leibovich, JB. Diabetes mellitus: Psychological issues in patient management. In JM Olefsky, RS Sherwin, Eds., *Diabetes Mellitus: Management and Complications,* New York: Churchill Livingstone, 1985, p. 353–376.

Jessor, R, Turbin, MS, Costa, FM. Protective factors in adolescent health behavior. *J Pers Soc Psychol* 75(3):788–800, 1998.

Katona, CLE, Manela, MV, Livingston, GA. Comorbidity with depression in older people: The Islington study. *Aging Ment Health* 1(1):57–61, 1997.

Kemeny, ME, Laudenslager, ML. Beyond stress: The role of individual difference factors in psychoneuroimmunology. *Brain Behav Imm* 13(2):73–75, 1999.

Kim, JY. A longitudinal study of interpersonal stress, major life events, and weekly stressors as predictors of pain and depression in fibromyalgia patients. (Doctoral dissertation, California School of Professional Psychology). *Diss Abstr Int* 61(2-B):1086, 2000.

Kludt, CJ. Effects of disease activity, neuroticism, and minor stress on pain perception in two immunologically distinct subgroups of patients with rheumatoid arthritis. (Doctoral dissertation, The Chicago Medical School, 2000). *Diss Abstr Int* 60(9-B):4892, 2000.

Knecht, S, Henningsen, H, Elbert, T, Flor, H, Hoeling, C, Pantev, C, Taub, E. Reorganizational and perceptual changes after amputation. *Brain* 119(4):1213–1219, 1996.

Koenig, H.G. *Aging and God: Spiritual Pathways to Mental Health in Midlife and Later Years.* New York: Haworth Press Inc., 534.

Lachman, ME, Weaver, SL. The sense of control as a moderator of social class differences in health and well-being. *J Pers Soc Psychol* 74(3):763–773, 1998.

Landreville, P, Gervais, PW. Psychotherapy for depression in older adults with disability: Where do we go from here? *Aging Ment Health* 1(3):197–208, 1997.

Langer, KG. Depression in disabling illness: Severity and patterns of self-reported symptoms in three groups. *J Geriatr Psychiatry Nurs* 7(2):121–128, 1994.

Longino, CF, Jr., Mittelmark, MB. Sociodemographic aspects. In J Sadavoy, LW Lazarus, Eds., *Comprehensive Review of Geriatric Psychology,* 2nd ed. Washington, DC: American Psychiatric Press, Inc., 1996.

Lopicic-Pericic, Z. Some aspects of nonverbal communication in psychotherapy of depressive patients. *Psychiatriki* 7(1):66–68, 1996.

Lundberg, U, Dohns, IE, Melin, B, Sandsjoe, L, Palmerud, G, Kadefors, R, Ekstroem, M, Parr, D. Psychophysiological stress responses, muscle tension, and neck and shoulder pain among supermarket cashiers. *J Occupat Health Psychol* 4(3):245–255, 1999.

McCarthy, ST., Ed. *Peripheral Vascular Disease in the Elderly.* New York: Churchill Livingstone, 1983.

McGarry, J. Hypnotic interventions in psychological and physiological aspects of amputation. *Aust J Clin Hypnotherapy Hypnosis* 14(1):7–12, 1993.

Melzack, R. Phantom limbs, the self, and the brain. *Can Psychol* 30(1):1–16, 1989.

Melzack, R. Pain and stress: Clues toward understanding chronic pain. In M Sabourin, F Craik, Eds., *Advances in Psychological Science, Vol. 2: Biological and Cognitive Aspects.* Hove, England: Psychology Press/Erlbaum, 1998, p. 63–85.

Melzack, R, Wall, P. *The Challenge of Pain.* London: Penguin Books, 352.

Mihalko, SL, McAuley, EL, Bane, SM. Self-efficacy and affective responses to acute exercise in middle-aged adults. *J Soc Behav Pers* 11(2):375–385, 1996.

Moxham, EG. The contribution of pain, nonrestorative sleep, depression, and stress to fatigue in fibromyalgia patients. (Doctoral dissertation, California School of Professional Psychology). *Diss Abstr Int* 60(4-B):1865, 1999.

Mullan, E, Markland, D. Variations in self-determinations across the stages of change for exercise in adults. *Motivation Emotion* 21(4):349–362, 1997.

New Lexicon Webster's Dictionary of the English Language. Bolander, DO, Bolander, A, Boak, SA, Buonocore, GF, Burke, SS, Castagno, JM, Churchill, JE, Jr, Izquierdo, M, Jewell, EJ, Lyon, R, Munoz, J, O'Reilly, M, Roth, RB, Sholtys, PM, Stodden, VL, Surprenant, DB and Vreeland, JAM, Eds. New York: Lexicon Publications, Inc., 1992.

Newsom, JT, Schulz, R. Social support as a mediator in the relation between functional status and quality of life in older adults. *Psychol Aging* 11(1):34–44, 1996.

Ormel, J, Kempen, GI, Pennix, BW, Brilman, EI, Beekman, AT, Van Sonderen, E. Chronic medical conditions and mental health in older people: Disability and psychosocial resources mediate specific mental health effects. *Psychol Med* 27(5):1065–1077, 1997.

Paterson, RJ, Neufeld, RWJ. What are my options: Influences of choice availability on stress and the perception of control. *J Res Pers* 29(2):145–167, 1995.

Pinel, JPJ. *Biopsychology*, 4th ed. Boston: Allyn and Bacon, 2000.

Rall, ML, Peskoff, FS, Byrne, JJ. The effects of information-giving behavior and gender on the perceptions of physicians: An experimental analysis. *Soc Behav Pers* 22(1):1–15, 1994.

Ratto, LL. *Coping with Being Physically Challenged.* New York: Rosen, 1991.

Roberts, RE, Kaplan, GA, Shema, SJ, Strawbridge, WJ. Prevalence and correlates of depression in an aging cohort: The Alameda County study. *J Gerontol: Series B: Psychol Sci Soc Sci* 52B(5):S252–S258, 1997.

Rybarczyk, B, Nyenhuis, DL, Nicholas, JJ, Cash, SM. Body image, perceived social stigma, and the prediction of psychosocial adjustment to leg amputation. *Rehabil Psychol* 40(2): 95–110, 1995.

Rybarczyk, B, Szymanski, L, Nicholas, JJ. Limb amputation. In R Frank, TR Elliott, Eds., *Handbook of Rehabilitation Psychology.* Washington, DC: American Psychological Association, 2000, p. 29–47.

Ryff, CD, Singer, B, Love, GD, Essex, MJ. Resilience in adulthood and later life: Defining features and dynamic processes. In J Lomranz, Ed., *Handbook of Aging and Mental Health: An Integrative Approach.* New York: Plenum Press, 1998, p. 69–96.

Snyder, RF. The relationship between learning styles, multiple intelligences, and academic achievement of high school students. *High School J* 83(2):11–20, 2000.

Stones, CR. Towards an attempt to anticipate sociopolitical change: A sociological perspective. *High School J* 75(4):203–208, 1992.

Thompson, SC, Nanni, C, Levine, A. Primary versus secondary and central versus consequence-related control in HIV-positive men. *J Pers Soc Psychol* 67(3):540–547, 1994.

Torff, B, Gardner, H. The vertical mind: The case for multiple intelligences. In M Anderson, Ed., *The Development of Intelligence. Studies in Developmental Psychology.* Hove, England: Psychology Press/Taylor and Francis, 1999, p. 139–159.

Tracey, DJ, Walker, JS, Carmody, JJ. Chronic pain: Neural basis and interactions with stress. In DT Kenny, JG Carlson, Eds., *Stress and Health: Research and Clinical Applications.* Amsterdam, Netherlands: Harwood Academic Publishers, 2000, p. 105–125.

Vedhara, K, Fox, JD, Wang, ECY. The measurement of stress-related immune dysfunction in psychoneuroimmunology. *Neurosci Biobehav Rev* 23(5):699–715, 1999.

Whitbourne, SK. Physical changes in the aging individual: Clinical implications. In IH Nordhus, GR Vandenbos, S Berg, P Fromholt, Eds., *Clinical Geropsychology.* Washington, DC: American Psychological Association, 1998, p. 79–108.

Williamson, GM. Restriction of normal activities among older adult amputees: The role of public self-consciousness. *J Clin Geropsychol* 1(3):229–242, 1995.

Williamson, GM, Schulz, R, Bridges, MW, Behan, AM. Social and psychological factors in adjustment to limb amputation. *J Soc Behav Pers* 9(5):249–268, 1994.

Wills, TA, DePaulo, BM. Interpersonal analysis of the help-seeking process. In CR Snyder, DR Forsyth, Eds., *Handbook of Social and Clinical Psychology: The Health Perspective, Vol. 162.* New York: Pergamon, 1991, p. 350–375.

Winett, RA. Developing more effective health-behavior programs: Analyzing the epidemiological and biological bases for activity and exercise programs. *Appl Prev Psychol* 7(4):209–224, 1998.

Index

Other Titles Available from the American Diabetes Association

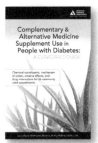

Complementary and Alternative Medicine (CAM) Supplement Use in People with Diabetes
by Laura Shane-McWhorter, PharmD, BCPS, FASCP, BC-ADM, CDE
Patients are often interested and excited by the prospects of complementary and alternative medicine supplementation. Keep yourself informed of this growing field, so you—and your patients—can make the safest, most effective decisions when it comes to CAM use.
Order no. 5433-01; Price $39.95

Therapy for Diabetes Mellitus and Related Disorders, 4th Edition
edited by Harold E. Lebovitz
Deliver proven treatments to your patients with this new edition of an essential book. Leading diabetes experts around the world provide a concise overview of the new advances in and an update on diabetes therapy, including glycemic control, type 2 diabetes prevention, diabetes in pregnancy, insulin pump therapy, and oral and cardiovascular disease.
Order no. 5402-04; Price $59.95

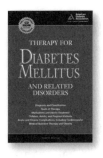

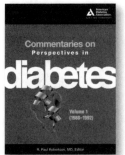

Commentaries on Perspectives in Diabetes
edited by R. Paul Robertson, MD
In this three-volume set, the original authors of many of the popular Perspectives in Diabetes articles published in the journal *Diabetes* revisit their original work and discuss what has changed over the past 18 years. Discover how the authors have given new life to their ideas, ensuring further and better development of new and effective therapies for diabetes.

Volume 1: Order no. 5430-01; Price $ 49.95
Volume 2: Order no. 5431-01; Price $ 49.95
Volume 3: Order no. 5432-01; Price $ 49.95
Complete Set: Order no. 6064-18; Price $104.95

Practical Insulin, 2nd Edition
by American Diabetes Association
This indispensable resource will give you the knowledge and data you need for initiating and maintaining insulin therapy in patients with type 1 or type 2 diabetes. Find fast, current, reliable information on insulin regimens, starting doses, correcting doses, insulin analogs, inhaled insulin, and matching insulin regimens to patients. With this easy reference guide, you can make improved glycemic control an attainable reality for your patients.

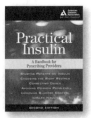

Order no. 5420-02; Price $7.95

About the American Diabetes Association

The American Diabetes Association is the nation's leading voluntary health organization supporting diabetes research, information, and advocacy. Its mission is to prevent and cure diabetes and to improve the lives of all people affected by diabetes. The American Diabetes Association is the leading publisher of comprehensive diabetes information. Its huge library of practical and authoritative books for people with diabetes covers every aspect of self-care— cooking and nutrition, fitness, weight control, medications, complications, emotional issues, and general self-care.

To order American Diabetes Association books: Call 1-800-232-6733 or log on to *http://store.diabetes.org*

To join the American Diabetes Association: Call 1-800-806-7801 or log on to *www. diabetes.org/membership*

For more information about diabetes or ADA programs and services: Call 1-800-342-2383. E-mail: AskADA@diabetes.org or log on to *www.diabetes.org*

To locate an ADA/NCQA Recognized Provider of quality diabetes care in your area: *www.ncqa.org/dprp*

To find an ADA Recognized Education Program in your area: Call 1-800-342-2383. *www.diabetes.org/for-health-professionals-and-scientists/recognition/edrecognition.jsp*

To join the fight to increase funding for diabetes research, end discrimination, and improve insurance coverage: Call 1-800-342-2383. *www.diabetes.org/advocacy-and-legalresources/advocacy.jsp*

To find out how you can get involved with the programs in your community: Call 1-800-342-2383. See below for program Web addresses.

- *American Diabetes Month:* educational activities aimed at those diagnosed with diabetes—month of November. *www.diabetes.org/communityprograms-and-localevents/ americandiabetesmonth.jsp*

- *American Diabetes Alert:* annual public awareness campaign to find the undiagnosed— held the fourth Tuesday in March. *www.diabetes.org/communityprograms-and-localevents/ americandiabetesalert.jsp*

- *American Diabetes Association Latino Initiative:* diabetes awareness program targeted to the Latino community. *www.diabetes.org/communityprograms-and-localevents/latinos.jsp*

- *African American Program:* diabetes awareness program targeted to the African American community. *www.diabetes.org/communityprograms-and-localevents/africanamericans.jsp*

- *Awakening the Spirit: Pathways to Diabetes Prevention & Control:* diabetes awareness program targeted to the Native American community. *www.diabetes.org/ communityprograms-and-localevents/nativeamericans.jsp*

To find out about an important research project regarding type 2 diabetes: *www.diabetes.org/diabetes-research/research-home.jsp*

To obtain information on making a planned gift or charitable bequest: Call 1-888-700-7029. *www.wpg.cc/stl/CDA/homepage/1,1006,509,00.html*

To make a donation or memorial contribution: Call 1-800-342-2383. *www.diabetes.org/support-the-cause/make-a-donation.jsp*

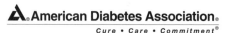
American Diabetes Association®
Cure • Care • Commitment®